T0214903

'Disorders of mood and personality are common after brain injury, and addressing these problems should be an integral part of neuropsychological rehabilitation. This edited volume provides descriptions and explanations of the current psychological therapies employed in good rehabilitation practice for survivors of acquired brain injury. Readers are provided with accounts of cognitive behaviour therapy, acceptance and commitment therapy, mindfulness, compassion focused therapy, positive psychology, attachment-based psychotherapies and integrative psychotherapy for holistic rehabilitation. The contributors are experts in their field, and any practitioner working in brain injury rehabilitation will recognise that this book is essential reading.'

–**Barbara A. Wilson**, *The Oliver Zangwill Centre,*
Ely, UK

'Despite dramatic advances in neuroscience over the past few decades, there is still no "cure" or effective biological treatment for many of the long-term neuropsychological consequences a lot of our patients face after an acquired brain injury. Covering a wide range of therapy models and techniques, *Psychological Therapies in Acquired Brain Injury* makes an important contribution to the field of long-term psychological care of patients who have suffered neurological injury or illness. Technically sound whilst simultaneously also hands-on and practical, this is an essential book for anyone interested in the application of psychotherapeutic approaches to caring for patients with acquired brain injury and their families.'

–**Rudi Coetzer**, *DClinPsy, Consultant Neuropsychologist*
and Head of Service, North Wales Brain Injury Service, UK

PSYCHOLOGICAL THERAPIES IN ACQUIRED BRAIN INJURY

The psychological impact of an acquired brain injury (ABI) can be devastating for both the person involved and their family. This book describes the different types of psychological therapies used to ameliorate psychological distress following ABI.

Each chapter presents a new therapeutic approach by experts in the area. Readers will learn about the key principles and techniques of the therapy alongside its application to a specific case following ABI. In addition, readers will gain insight into which approach may be most beneficial to whom as well as those where there may be additional challenges. Covering a wide array of psychological therapies, samples range from more historically traditional approaches to those more recently developed.

Psychological Therapies in Acquired Brain Injury will be of great interest to clinicians and researchers working in brain injury rehabilitation, as well as practitioners, researchers and students of psychology, neuropsychology and rehabilitation.

Giles N. Yeates is Editor of the journal and book series *Neuro-Disability & Psychotherapy*, in addition to the Brain Injury book series (Routledge Books). As a clinical neuropsychologist in community neurorehabilitation, his clinical work and research focuses on the innovation of psychological therapies and support of relationships following acquired brain injury, and he has published widely on these topics. Dr Yeates is currently innovating the use of Tai Ji in neurorehabilitation.

Fiona Ashworth is a clinical psychologist and senior lecturer who has worked with people with acquired brain injuries for over 20 years. She trained as a clinical psychologist at Oxford University and went on to work at the Oliver Zangwill Centre for Neuropsychological Rehabilitation where her passion for working psychotherapeutically with people with acquired brain injuries began. She continues her clinical work alongside researching psychological distress and its amelioration following acquired brain injury.

Current Issues in Neuropsychology

Series Editor: Jon Evans

University of Glasgow, Glasgow, UK

Current Issues in Neuropsychology is a series of edited books that reflect the state-of-the-art in areas of current and emerging interest in the psychological study of brain damage, behaviour and cognition.

Each volume is tightly focused on a particular topic, with chapters contributed by international experts. The editors of individual volumes are leading figures in their areas and provide an introductory overview of the field.

Each book will reflect an issue, area of uncertainty or controversy, with contributors providing a range of views on the central topic. Examples include the question of whether technology can enhance, support or replace impaired cognition, and how best to understand, assess and manage alcohol related brain damage.

Published titles in the series:

Assistive Technology for Cognition
Edited by Brian O'Neill and Alex Gillespie

Alcohol and the Adult Brain
Jenny Svanberg, Adrienne Withall, Brian Draper and Stephen Bowden

Degenerative Disorders of the Brain
Darren R. Hocking, John L. Bradshaw and Joanne Fielding

Psychological Therapies in Acquired Brain Injury
Edited by Giles N. Yeates and Fiona Ashworth

PSYCHOLOGICAL THERAPIES IN ACQUIRED BRAIN INJURY

*Edited by Giles N. Yeates
and Fiona Ashworth*

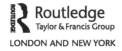
Routledge
Taylor & Francis Group

LONDON AND NEW YORK

First published 2020
by Routledge
2 Park Square, Milton Park, Abingdon, Oxon OX14 4RN

and by Routledge
52 Vanderbilt Avenue, New York, NY 10017

Routledge is an imprint of the Taylor & Francis Group, an informa business

British Library Cataloguing-in-Publication Data
A catalogue record for this book is available from the British Library

Library of Congress Cataloging-in-Publication Data
A catalog record for this book has been requested

ISBN: 978-1-138-58124-1 (hbk)
ISBN: 978-1-138-58126-5 (pbk)
ISBN: 978-0-429-50679-6 (ebk)

Typeset in Bembo
by Apex CoVantage, LLC

CONTENTS

FIGURES

Graphs

TABLES

EDITORS' FOREWORD

Psychotherapy within neurorehabilitation and its' emerging evidence has come a long way in the last 50 years, and we are thankful to Kurt Goldstein, Yehuda Ben-Yishay and George Prigatano for the inception and ensuing foundations they laid. When attempting to reduce psychological distress and improve wellbeing for individuals with neurological conditions, what works for whom continues to be an intricate and complex affair for clinicians to untangle. Indeed, this complexity that marks each novel encounter between a clinician and a person with a neurological condition who has a unique combination of physical, cognitive, emotional and social strengths and needs is a key factor in drawing many of us to this specialist field and keeping us here for a full career. Alongside this clinical experience, the challenge for research is to ensure that the people we work with, the full heterogeneous range of people who have suffered traumatic brain injury or stroke, are represented in studies examining new and existing therapies. Exclusion approaches that aim to optimise homogeneity under a broad diagnostic label such as traumatic brain injury result in findings that can often feel too adrift from the complexity and diversity of our clinical encounters. Promising alternatives such as sampling brain injury sub-groups that are homogenous around a particular deficit, single case experimental designs and qualitative studies informed by deep, rich epistemological sampling strategies are yet to become sufficiently commonplace in the literature. Accordingly, our knowledge base as clinicians is as dependent not just on large n samples but on evocative case study reports of specific pieces of psychotherapeutic work with particular presentations, illuminating diverse intervention orientations and the different fruits they yield. We hope this edited volume has yielded many resources of this kind for our readers.

Working in the field, we are all too aware of the need to practice a much more eclectic approach to psychological interventions with our clients. With a holistic perspective, we formulate globally then hone into the specific and then back out to the wider perspective again, whilst keeping a keen focus on the human being at the centre of this process and considering how the neurological condition impacts on them and how we can best work together to ameliorate difficulties. As Bernard Beitman put it, 'Psychotherapy challenges us to comprehend the ethereal mind interacting with the earthy brain' (Beitman, 2007, Foreword). No more so than in our client group. This book is borne from that very need – a need to work out how best we can support the client sitting in front of us. This book aims to encompass the richness and variety of psychological approaches currently being used with people with neurological conditions. Each chapter covers a specific approach representing established and contemporary traditions that focus on individual, couples, family and group formats and define the relationship of the injured mind and body differentially as the scope of intervention. We wanted to consider not which approach might be best, as this would be naïve, but consider where one approach might fit best for a particular client, as well as highlighting the richness of multimodal perspectives that are emerging within clinical practice. Conversations with clinicians in the field reflected a need to better understand the specific types of approaches people are using, with a focus on understanding what the approaches are, their core elements, how they are applied to those with neurological conditions, what the evidence is telling us, for which particular clients might that approach be better suited in our group and where might it be contra-indicated or present significant challenges. In addition, considerations for adaptations are discussed as well as therapists' reflections on their weddedness to the particular approach they are drawn too. Finally, each approach draws these elements together through a case vignette demonstrating the therapy approach in action in this client group, including the client's/s' voice/s. We believe this book provides a rich source of information on the application of different psychological approaches to psychological distress in neurological conditions. As such, when you as the clinician reader encounters a new and unique combination of physical, cognitive, emotional and social needs with the people you so importantly support, we trust you'll find an idea, example and principle from one of these chapters that will feel useful. We are proud as editors to claim that the diversity of such presentations is matched by the diversity of ideas, approaches and foundational assumptions presented in this book. We hope this book will offer both experienced and novel readers insight and understanding into the diversity of the approaches being used and will aid them in their clinical practice.

Giles N. Yeates and Fiona Ashworth

Reference

Beitman, B. (2007). Foreword. In K. Grawe (Ed.), *Neuropsychotherapy: How the neurosciences inform effective psychotherapy* (p. XIII). New York: Taylor and Francis.

ACKNOWLEDGEMENTS

As the editors we are indebted to those who have provided contributions to each chapter and recognise much of the tireless and pioneering work that is going on across communities by our colleagues. This book has been in the making for a significant period of time; during the making of our labour of love, life has thrown challenges at us, and we are thankful to those who have been patient with us, including our chapter authors and our publishers and series editor Professor Jon Evans; also, thanks go to Ste Weatherhead for his pivotal role during early conversations and planning for this book.

1

APPLICATION OF THE COGNITIVE BEHAVIOURAL APPROACH TO ENHANCING EMOTIONAL OUTCOMES FOLLOWING ACQUIRED BRAIN INJURY (ABI)

Fergus Gracey, Peter Smits, Pieter du Toit, Jessica Fish and Kate Psaila

Introduction

This chapter presents the conceptual background to CBT and its application following ABI. We summarise our trans-diagnostic cognitive-behavioural model aimed at enabling the therapist to understand and engage more deeply with someone's lived experience following ABI and to aid collaborative identification of interventions. Along the way, we outline our view of what 'CBT' entails and the outcomes we are seeking to achieve with people with brain injury. We provide a brief description of the key therapeutic activities and map these to our clinical model, finally illustrating diversity of application with two cases.

Theoretical and practical background to cognitive behavioural therapies

Cognitive behavioural therapy (CBT) is now ubiquitous in clinical psychological practice and mental health services, for some seeming synonymous with evidence-based practice (occasionally regardless of strength of evidence relating to a specific disorder, condition or patient). The term is also often used as if denoting a single, specific form of practice: 'CBT'. However, the very wide range of CBTs applicable for different clinical challenges and delivered in different service contexts indicate that CBT is not one thing. Nor is it, in our view, simply a case of being different depending on which emotional disorder it is pointed at. Corrie and Lane (2015), in their book on supervision in CBT highlight multiple continua against which we can rate our style of CBT practice, spanning straight behavioural through to fully cognitive, minimally second wave to fully third wave, protocol-based through to formulation-led, etc. We have previously argued that in practice working with those with more complex challenges, and in particular working in ABI, 'CBT' may well comprise a range of interventions drawn from behavioural, cognitive, disorder-specific, transdiagnostic and third wave as arrived at through formulation with the client and aligned to their values and aspirations (Ownsworth & Gracey, 2017).

Despite this diversity, there are theoretical and practical commonalities across CB approaches which we perceive as being fundamental to CB practice in ABI. Theoretical commonalities include:

- A focus on personal meaning (as articulated in beliefs, assumptions and other forms of mental representation) as underlying a given issue: "The concentration on exploring the meaning of events throughout the course of therapy . . . should be encouraged" (Beck, Rush, Shaw, & Emery, 1979, p. 33). We are heavily influenced by Teasdale and Barnard's (1993) distinction between propositional and implicational meanings, with the latter being the target for change as implicational representations map rich, subjective, 'felt sense' of self-in-context.
- The notion that underlying meaning elicited in a type, or types, of situation is reciprocally associated with cognitive, behavioural, emotional and physiological processes, such that change in one domain might result in changes in other domains.
- The likelihood that some aspects of the cognitive, behavioural, emotional and physiological responses that arise in given situations might be related to personal historical factors, such as early experiences.
- There is a causal chain of processes linking responses in 'trigger' situations to longer term maintenance or deepening of problems (for example where the initial response in turn becomes a further 'trigger').
- Cognitive processes are not fixed, but dynamically shift according to the nature of currently active meanings and emotional processes (for example, a feeling of lack of energy might trigger a spiral of negative self-focused rumination, once ruminating the person may become less able to think flexibly, problem solve or make more nuanced, less black and white interpretations of events, and memory retrieval becomes more over-general and negatively biased; see Mansell, Harvey, Watkins, & Shafran, 2008).
- It is relatively structured and time limited with the aim of achieving one or more specific aims identified by the client.
- There is a focus on the client practicing between sessions, as well as within sessions, in order to generate the desired shifts in meanings, emotions or behaviours.
- The general orientation is one of curiosity and exploration (originally described by Beck as 'collaborative empiricism'), where the therapist works alongside the client rather than taking the 'expert role'.

There are also a number of practical and structural commonalities across CBTs:

- The therapist informs the person about the principles of the CBT being used (providing information) and links the information to examples and practice in session (socialising to the model).
- The therapist fosters a collaborative rapport with the client within which new meanings can be identified and explored (typically using a model which summarises the key processes pertaining to a particular clinical problem area), allowing the client to begin to reflect on and organise their subjective experiences.
- The therapist wonders with the client about whether this formulation might help to identify areas to change in order to move towards their goals.
- This collaborative and reflective process sets the foundation for introducing specific techniques associated with that model or approach to treatment that address the core processes assumed to be generating vulnerability to, or maintenance of, the problem.
- Techniques are explained and practiced in session, and the client asked to reflect on their experience of using the technique and what changes or effects they think it might have.
- Therapy proceeds with developing and deepening specific practices, for example: identifying unhelpful thinking patterns in session then as homework, developing different ways of responding to these thinking patterns first in session then as homework, practicing the acts of catching and reflecting on unhelpful thinking until it becomes increasingly automatic.
- Whilst the targets are often cognitive in nature (thoughts, images, assumptions, beliefs, thinking styles such as catastrophising or personalising, processes such as rumination), interventions will necessarily involve behaviour change – manipulating behaviour in a specific trigger situation to explicitly test things out ('behavioural experiments': see McGrath et al., 2004).
- Every endeavour should be made to work with the client in emotionally 'hot' situations (evoked in a clinic-based session, in everyday life, at home, in relationships, or involving significant others; Beck et al., 1979).
- This may involve working directly with emotion (for example using a calming or compassionate image, increasing engagement in pleasurable activities and attending more fully to positive or other emotional experiences).
- Therapy endings are carefully planned to include a 'blueprint' for predicting and managing set-backs, ensuring continued change/consolidation post therapy and might include follow-up or booster sessions.

Application of CBTs when working in acquired brain injury

Working with people with ABI means engaging with a very diverse range of presenting needs and challenges, responded to in diverse ways by individuals with varied profiles of functioning. There is unlikely to be a single model that fits all.

Nevertheless, we have over some years of exploring and adapting our approach, identified some key processes we think can be applied transdiagnostically, that are reflected also in research evidence (Gracey, Evans, & Malley, 2009; Gracey, Ford, & Psaila, 2015; Ownsworth & Gracey, 2017; Shields, Ownsworth, O'Donovan, & Fleming, 2016) which we draw upon in the remainder of this chapter. Here we cover in turn: targets for change, the model to guide formulation, intervention components and adaptations and contra-indications.

Targets for therapeutic change

We conceive three overlapping ways in which CB approaches can be applied to improve wellbeing and reduce distress, where necessary, following brain injury.

1   Some aspect of the ABI, or life after ABI, is a trigger for underlying beliefs and assumptions to be activated, in line with the traditional view of cognitive models of emotional disorders. Here an individual might present predominantly with a single clear emotional disorder (perhaps with some variation depending on the individual, their acquired deficits and circumstances). Specific evidence-based cognitive behavioural therapy based on the appropriate diagnosis-specific model might be applicable, albeit with modifications to address acquired cognitive or other difficulties.

2   The new and challenging circumstances that arise post-ABI result in a mix of subjective experiences and symptoms such as disinhibited or uncharacteristic emotional reactions, altered sense of identity, or sense of loss of self, unhelpful coping (including 'denial of disability'), low self-esteem (and low self-efficacy) and absence of (opportunities for) experiences that might contribute to new meaning-making. Research in to transdiagnostic factors has identified threat to self and emotion dysregulation as two common underlying processes across depression, anxiety and stress post TBI (Shields et al., 2016). For this group, we have developed two models, and related intervention targets and processes, based on the centrality of altered sense of personal and social identity to maintaining unwanted outcomes (Gracey, Evans et al., 2009; Gracey et al., 2015).

3   In both these cases, unless the acquired deficits are relatively mild, life post-ABI is likely to be radically changed, and individuals may need support to move beyond resolution of disconnection with self, or threat to self, to achieving sense of purpose, finding positive meanings, (re)connecting with self and others in everyday life (Ownsworth & Gracey, 2017). A broader conceptualisation of 'outcomes' than resumption of activity or reduction of 'symptoms' is required; one that allows for entry into the unknown, to be open to exploration and discovery of new meanings that may arise despite, or perhaps because of, the challenges being faced (for example as described in models of Post-Traumatic Growth: Tedeschi & Calhoun, 2004; Powell,

Ekin-Wood, & Collin, 2007; Silva, Ownsworth, Shields, & Fleming, 2011). Intervention approaches may be more concerned with finding the conditions in which someone can explore and develop new and valued meanings in life. Whilst CB techniques (such as 'possibility dreaming': Mooney & Padesky, 2000) could be used to support 'constructive' work (Gracey, Brentnall, & Megoran, 2009) there is a growing body of evidence concerning approaches drawn from other schools of thought (e.g., positive psychology: Cullen et al., 2018; arts: Ellis-Hill et al., 2015; Baylan, Swann-Price, Peryer, & Quinn, 2016; and mindfulness: Bédard et al., 2014), which could feature as part of a broader constructive rehabilitative endeavour.

A transdiagnostic cognitive behavioural approach to working in ABI

In our work over some years to improve attention to subjective needs in rehabilitation, and improve CBT practice in ABI, we have developed two models from which specific interventions can be identified:

- The transdiagnostic cognitive behavioural model of adaptation post-ABI (Gracey et al., 2015) describes the ways in which immediate understandable momentary emotional reactions in the context of changed life post ABI can be made sense of in terms of 'threats to self', echoing Goldstein's (1952) description of the psychological consequences of ABI. The model distinguishes between a number of linked cognitive-behavioural processes. These include pre-injury factors (including assumptions and rules for living, coping styles) that might pre-dispose someone to experience certain post-injury challenges as a particular 'threat-to-self', the actual changes someone faces, in-the-moment threat reactions triggered when faced with challenges, effects of self-regulatory deficits and longer term meaning-making and coping patterns (e.g., avoidance, emotion-focused, substance misuse, attempts at mental or emotional control, acceptance) that ultimately further influence that person's everyday circumstances. We broke the full model down into a more accessible 'vicious daisy' as a potential tool for facilitating collaborative formulation, presented (with permission) in Figure 1.1.
- The Y-Shaped model (Gracey, Evans et al., 2009; Ownsworth & Gracey, 2017) describes the conditions under which rehabilitation activity and identity change can be brought together in a relatively structured process to help reduce sense of discrepancy and disconnection, and in time develop personal and social (re)connections and new ways of being in the world. The emphasis is on progressive cycles of exploration linking as necessary with rehabilitation activities in personally valued roles or contexts. The most recent version of the model is influenced by the phenomenological model of wellbeing described by Galvin and Todres (2011) and observations working on a trial of

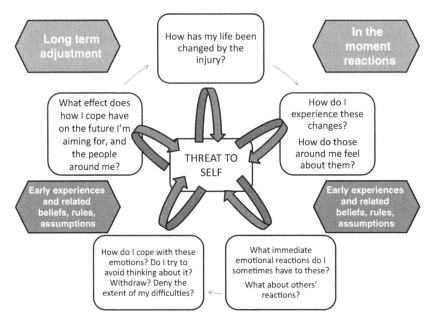

FIGURE 1.1 The 'threat-to-self vicious daisy' model providing a simplified version of the transdiagnostic cognitive-behavioural model based on Gracey et al. (2015), adapted with permission from Routledge Press.

an Arts and Health intervention for confidence post-stroke (Ellis-Hill et al., 2015): ensuring that the contextual conditions are right for 'stepping into the unknown' and creatively discovering new insights and meanings.

Key intervention components

Figure 1.2 maps examples of cognitive-behavioural or rehabilitation interventions that might be applicable to some of the 'petals' of the vicious daisy. This is not an exhaustive list, but merely illustrates the way in which client and therapist creativity coupled with the existing literature on cognitive behavioural and other therapies can be combined to find helpful techniques to address processes maintaining sense of threat to identity. In the following we provide a summary outlining the general process of therapy, although noting that again, for some, there might be a need to modify according to needs.

Psychoeducation and socialisation to the model – subjective sense of identity change and responses to it

Socialisation to the model is an early task in the process of CBT that enables the client and therapist to work collaboratively together through therapy. It can start with information provision, although the process of finding everyday examples

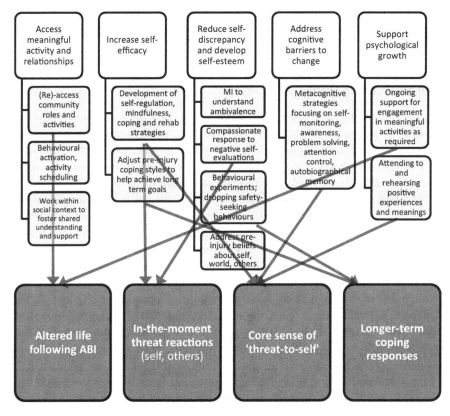

FIGURE 1.2 Domains and types of intervention mapped on to 'petals' of the threat-to-self vicious daisy

illustrating the core features of the cognitive behavioural approach being provided is more in keeping with the collaborative approach of CBT, and also models the approach itself.

In terms of modification of this socialisation process for ABI, we find that discussions about pre-post-injury changes, including changes to sense of self, can provide a useful starting point. It is important to emphasise that negative emotions perform a function and are understandable as 'normal' human reactions to challenging situations. The Y-shaped model and threat vicious daisy can readily be applied as tools for supporting discussion of identity change with people with BI and their families (Gracey et al., 2017). The models can helpfully illustrate how someone might be 'stuck' battling with trying to manage this sense of changed identity, disconnection or 'discrepancy' (within themselves and/or with others). They can also help to illustrate how completely understandable ways of reacting to specific triggers can over time lead to unhelpful patterns of coping that further disadvantage the person in their quest for continuity in sense of identity, meaning making and sense of purpose. Using these diagrams (or simplified versions of them) can also support cognitive and communication issues that might otherwise be a barrier to socialisation and collaboration.

Exploring the underlying core 'threats to self' in response to momentary triggers

As previously discussed, the provisional transdiagnostic CBT model and Y-Shaped models we previously described propose that the central meanings underpinning emotional problems post-BI relate to 'threat to self'. The Y-Shaped model describes such experiences as those that denote a sense of self that is at odds with a desired or valued sense of self (often seen as equivalent to pre-injury sense of self).

The first step in therapy following from these models is to focus on identifying and 'formulating' what occurs in very specific emotionally 'hot' moments, tracking moment-to-moment changes in thoughts, feelings, behaviours and physiological changes (as best the person can report, as observed if in a real-world context, or as recorded using a heart rate monitor or biofeedback device). Emotionally salient moments are seen as the substrate of broader, enduring self-representations in a number of models of identity (see, for example, Ownsworth & Haslam, 2016). Often people will have very quick, possibly disinhibited emotional responses which they can only really make sense of after the event. It is possible that the nonconscious 'quick and dirty' route (LeDoux, 2003) to threat has been activated, so conscious awareness of the response can only occur through noticing internal physiological changes (difficult for many of us, even more so after a brain injury) or becoming aware of one's behaviour through feedback and post-event reflection. It is often the case that close observation (or reports of those present at the time) are needed to help ascertain the moment at which the emotional 'threat' response was triggered and the nature of the behavioural manifestation of threat (e.g., anxious agitation and distractibility, aggression, defeated withdrawal or passivity, tearfulness).

As with many CBT approaches, practice at self-monitoring using structured homework may be helpful. In ABI this could take whatever form is deemed most appropriate and won't necessarily be traditional 'five column technique' for identifying and responding to negative automatic thoughts. Learning mindfulness meditation techniques, particularly body scan, can be of assistance in helping to tune in to and stay with physiological changes, and mindfulness of breathing in session can help provide insight into 'background' repeating patterns of thinking or meaning. In-vivo observation is also helpful. We have also used heart rate monitors and a wearable camera to enhance this aspect of therapy where impairments might present a barrier (Brindley, Bateman, & Gracey, 2011).

Following on from identification of threat reactions, any number of self-regulatory strategies could be applied depending on the specific type of threat activation and emotional experience. Simple resonant breathing or 'on the spot arousal reduction' techniques can be used to help reduce autonomic nervous system arousal (we often use a metaphor of 'putting the brakes on' for this type of strategy). Relaxing or compassionate images could also be developed and applied. Mindfulness can foster a more accepting, curious approach to mental events; responding to whatever arises without trying to change it can be of help for some (the metaphor of 'pressing the clutch down' rather than applying the brakes can be useful here). Increasing in complexity, the person could learn to apply traditional thought challenging or reframing strategies, problem solving or goal management techniques to help 'catch' a quickly developing threat reaction and take alternative action. Obtaining ratings of strength of subjective experience (e.g., of arousal, anxiety, a sense of 'not being me') can help structure a more nuanced appreciation of subtle variation in experience itself helpful in supporting self-regulation abilities.

Linking subjective identity change, meaning and rehabilitation goals through behavioural experiments

Our experience led us to focus on the unhelpful assumptions associated with 'threat' triggering moments as a key cognitive target, rather than negative automatic thoughts. Therefore, having first focused on what occurs in very specific 'hot' moments, the next step is to extend conceptualisation to longer term attempts to reduce threat to self. For example, a client may experience an increase in anxiety and self-consciousness, feeling muddled and stressed when attempting to prepare a family meal. If a well-meaning family member offers to help this might elicit a snappy, aggressive response. Assumptions might then be identifiable that link these specific moments with broader adjustment and adaptation, for example 'If I can't manage cooking a meal for my family, then I'm on the scrap heap', 'If I'm angry with my family it just shows I'm not fit to be a parent, I'm so ashamed, they'd be better off without me'. These assumptions may really help to make sense of how, over time, the client tends to avoid the kitchen completely, further feeling more disconnected from his identity, to the point when he decides he is going to make a big effort to cook an elaborate meal, with insufficient planning and disastrous consequences. The outcome of either avoiding, or attempting something too complex with inadequate planning, will feed into the longer-term sense of life being different post-injury, and further confirmation of fears and deepening of threats to self.

Assumption-based interventions flow naturally from this, making explicit links between underlying meanings, behavioural responses and attempts to 'seek safety' by reducing threat to self. Behavioural experiments can be developed from asking the question 'how could we test this out', 'what would happen if . . . ?' or 'how could we explore this?'. A number of examples are provided in the literature (Dewar & Gracey, 2007; Gracey, Brentnall et al., 2009; Gracey, Malley et al., 2009; Gracey, Oldham, & Kritzinger, 2007; McGrath et al., 2004; Judd & Wilson, 2005). Embedding behavioural experiments in rehabilitation activities can be an excellent way for individuals to experience shifts in their experience of themselves, initially in specific situations, then across new and potentially expanding aspects of their life. In addition, it provides a means by which the person can be engaged in thinking about strategy use as a tool to enhance reconnection with self, very helpful when strategy use itself is a trigger for provoking unhelpful assumptions ('If I use a strategy the brain injury has beaten me', 'If others see me using a strategy they'll think I'm weak'). New assumptions might arise that can be built upon (e.g., 'If I pick a simpler meal and take time to plan, using my goal management framework, then I can prepare a meal for my family, I can be that person again, that "provider"'). So post-experiment reflections can focus equally on 'what I learnt about "me"' and 'what I learnt about strategies that might be helpful'. Developed and delivered well, behavioural experiments provide a safe 'win, win' scenario in which both client and therapist can only learn. In our experience, having worked systematically in this way over a number of sessions, towards the end of therapy clients often describe a sense of being ready to try things out in life, experiment and not worry too much if things go wrong, as this can be learned from.

It should be noted that for many, engaging in behavioural experiments might initially 'expose' the person to their underlying fears (e.g., 'everyone will laugh at me', 'no one will want to know me') with a risk of activating broader negative beliefs and associated emotional and behavioural reactions. Therefore, it is important to have a clear formulation underlying the behavioural experiment which allows prediction of certain meanings and emotions being elicited. If certain behaviours that are a target in a behavioural experiment serve as 'safety-seeking behaviours', dropping these will inevitably lead to an increase in anticipatory or in situ sense of threat to self. Where someone's ability to cope with or regulate emotions is not strong or is risky (e.g., frequent aggressive outbursts, use of drugs or alcohol, withdrawal from rehabilitation or social support, negative self-focused rumination, suicidality), this will need addressing first. It is possible that cognitive deficits might not only enhance negative emotional reactions but might also have positive effects. For example, we have noticed some distractible clients can be easily 'cued' out of ruminative or negative perseverative thinking to good effect. A recent study found those with good working memory who ruminated fair worse emotionally than those with poor working memory (Ownsworth, Gooding, & Beadle, 2019).

Finding a new way of being in the world

Following this phase, intervention might proceed to the process of positive adaptation in which people discover for themselves new ways of being in the world. The Y-Shaped model describes the constructive process of building a 'new me' that follows after addressing and reducing the unhelpful ways of avoiding 'threat to self' in which people might be stuck. As described earlier, a recent revision of the model further emphasises the importance of the context around the individual in providing opportunities, or creating the circumstances needed, for constructive change (Ownsworth & Gracey, 2017).

What works for whom: adaptations and contra-indications

There have been a number of published reviews of psychological therapies including CBTs covering treatment or prevention of depression (Gertler, Tate, & Cameron, 2015; Hackett, Anderson, House, & Halteh, 2008; Stalder-Lüthy, Messerli-Bürgy, Hofer, Frischknecht, Znoj, & Barth, 2013), anxiety (Soo & Tate, 2007) and other common emotional consequences across ABI (Ownsworth & Gracey, 2017; Waldron, Casserly, & O'Sullivan, 2013). The diversity of findings suggests no clear, robust evidence for 'CBT', from which conclusions about 'what works for whom' can be drawn. Some individual studies do appear to show positive effects (e.g., Simpson, Tate, Whiting, & Cotter, 2011; Arundine et al., 2012; Bédard et al., 2014; Hsieh et al., 2012; Thomas, Walker, MacNiven, Haworth, & Lincoln, 2013). Waldron et al. (2013) concluded that CBT appears most effective when the treatment model/approach and primary outcome are specific and aligned. A tentative conclusion can be made that, depending on intervention targets and goals, it may be better to: attend carefully to neuropsychological needs and adapt sessions as necessary (Bradbury, Christensen, Lau, Ruttan, Arundine, & Green, 2008); address coping, meaning making and hope for the future (Simpson, Tate, Whiting, & Cotter, 2011); and foster stress reduction, mindful noticing of mental events, disruption of ruminative thinking, and compassionate acceptance of oneself (Bédard et al., 2014).

Issues with awareness can be a significant barrier to progress with rehabilitation. Supported feedback approaches have the best evidence for helping people (see Schmidt, Fleming, Ownsworth, & Lannin, 2013; Schmidt, Lannin, Fleming, & Ownsworth, 2011) and in a survey of approaches adopted by therapists, BE's were reported as commonly used to work with awareness issues (Judd & Wilson, 2005). Within our model, problems with awareness can be helpfully formulated where it serves a function of protecting against threat to self in the moment or over the longer term (Ownsworth et al., 2007; Yeates, Henwood, Gracey, & Evans, 2007). Identifying situations under which the person more strongly denies difficulties, or is more amenable to reflect on them, might help give some clues as to triggers for threat-based denial of difficulties, or conditions that support awareness, which can be built upon in formulation and intervention. Involvement of others (family, other professionals or rehabilitation staff) may well be required.

In the previous example we have highlighted the key features that might present in a typical clinical case, with mention of adaptations for cognitive limitations (by integrating therapy with past or current rehabilitation, modifying materials). However, further adaptation may be required depending on cognitive, communication, emotional or behavioural factors (see Gracey et al., 2015; Ownsworth & Gracey, 2017; Gallagher, McLeod, & McMillan, 2019). The approach is likely to be most accessible to those with less impaired intellectual or communication difficulties. CBT itself lends itself well to supporting people with cognitive difficulties through providing a structured approach to sessions, with application of between-session behavioural practice. Generally speaking, greater cognitive or communication impairment might require a more behavioural approach, however, seeking to understand and engage with subjective experience should not be neglected. Additional adaptations can be applied depending on need, for example working collaboratively with communication partners, simplifying therapy materials and emphasising the behavioural interventions more, and including standard compensatory strategies (such as reminder-setting, using periodic cues or alerts, including homework tasks within any external memory and planning system) for managing the impact of cognitive impairments. There is an increasing role of technology being applied to support these strategies that can also be considered.

As previously mentioned, some individuals may have additional emotional vulnerabilities, possibly predating the ABI, which make work involving dropping coping behaviours that protect against perceived threats to self potentially challenging. Where the formulation indicates a lack of skills in managing strong emotional reactions effectively, work to enhance self-regulatory skills may be required. For some, working according to this full model may be too risky initially. Discussion of intervention pros and cons should be collaborative, with reference to the formulation and with relevant close others or family members. A 'goal management' approach to support decision making might be helpful here, and clinical risk assessment may well be warranted.

Currently in the UK, the National Health Service (NHS) aims to provide accessible, evidence-based interventions, mainly cognitive-behavioural self-help techniques and CBT, for people with anxiety and depression through Improving Access to Psychological Therapy (IAPT) services (Clark, 2011). There is a drive to make this service accessible to people with long-term conditions (LTC, such as chronic obstructive pulmonary disease, diabetes), with an estimated 40% of IAPT service users presenting with a co-morbid LTC. Training and adaptations have been recognised as necessary for clinicians working with these client groups (National Collaborating Centre for Mental Health, 2018). However, ABI and stroke are not mentioned within this guidance. IAPT is a stepped care model with Step 1 comprising of assessment, psychoeducation and signposting to other services, Step 2 (low intensity interventions) involving supported self-help, including computerised CBT (cCBT) and psycho-educational groups, and Step 3 (high intensity) featuring face-to-face therapeutic interventions with individuals or couples (National Institute for Health and Clinical Evidence, 2011; Kneebone, 2015). There are a small number of examples where community neurorehabilitation/neuropsychology services and IAPT services have developed shared pathways to improve access to psychological therapies for people with ABIs (King, Pimm, & Tyerman, 2014). Our experience is that some are able to benefit from this service, where IAPT clinicians liaise with the psychologist in the neurorehabilitation services. Based on our experience, the clients most likely to benefit are those (described in section 3a, and with case 'Mr E' in section 4) with a single clear emotional disorder and some adaptations needed, who can access and make use of specific strategies or techniques. Where appropriate we make recommendations for a face to face consultation and a high intensity intervention, providing background information about the neuropsychological sequelae and any recommended adaptations. Clients can benefit from the regular structured intervention, alongside their other neurorehabilitation interventions. Low intensity interventions may have too many barriers for people to access, arising from demands on abilities to be able to engage in a self-directed intervention, although there is some evidence of potential for people post stroke to engage in a supported cCBT intervention (Simblett et al., 2017). Some clients also require support with the self-referral process. As the severity of the presenting problems increase, more specialist intervention is likely to be required, with an increasing need for clinical neuropsychology involvement, explicitly linking therapy with rehabilitation, and involving family or others in the person's system. The weak (for stroke) and mixed (for TBI) evidence base for CBT, should be held in mind and the assumption that 'CBT is an evidence-based intervention' for ABI in the context of the IAPT service model should be avoided.

Case examples

In this section we present two case examples briefly illustrating the ways in which the model can be applied to guide cognitive behavioural intervention.

Case 1: Mr E – social anxiety

Mr E is a 22-year-old man who suffered multiple traumas, including a moderately severe traumatic brain injury, following a traffic accident. A few years prior to his own accident, Mr E witnessed his father having a stroke, the aftermath of which included family tensions and elevated anxiety, including panic attacks.

In early post-acute rehabilitation and whilst likely still emerging from PTA, Mr E was unable to remember what he had said to others during visits (for example his friends), from which he developed worry and anxiety that he might have said something stupid or wrong. After discharge, this fear generalised to other social situations, despite his memory having improved significantly.

Mr E became afraid of situations in which people could ask how he was doing. This could, for example, be a sudden meeting in the street or when he was entering the office building of his former employer and thereby would be the centre of attention of the whole office staff. The threat response elicited in this kind of situation was characterised by feelings of panic and depersonalisation, which further reminded him of his confusion during his PTA phase, causing further fear and anxiety. Consistent with the model of Clark and Wells (1995) he became conscious of going red with self-consciousness, and with struggling to find his words. Mr E became convinced that others would find his blushing and stuttering particularly strange and over time he did not dare go shopping at the shopping centre or to return to his former job. Initial assessment indicated elevated emotional symptoms and a passive rather than active, problem-oriented coping style. The formulation of this cycle of in-the-moment and longer-term responses is provided in Figure 1.3.

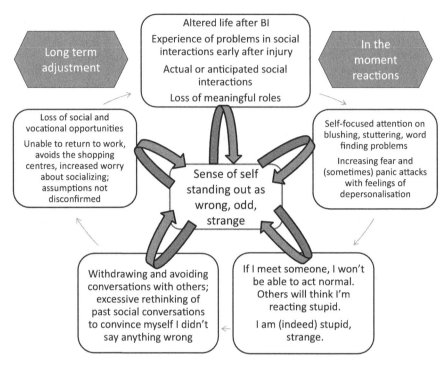

FIGURE 1.3 Vicious daisy formulation for Mr E, illustrating how in-the-moment anxieties about social interactions deepened and generalised over time leading to further reduction of social participation and increase in anxiety symptoms

Mr E's goal was to return to his former job as a package deliverer, which was supported by his former boss. This job gave him some self-confidence in a difficult period in his life (as a result of the problems with his father and his own panic attacks). The treatment started with education about physical reactions and sensations that arise as a response to a threatening situation. After this we conducted attention training (based on Wells, 1997) in order to help redirect self-focused attention (on blushing and stuttering) to the conversation and to improve his self-efficacy, which he also practiced at home. We prepared sentences he could use in a conversation if people asked about his health and practiced these in session using role-play. Because Mr E was insecure about (what others thought about) his work skills we did some cognitive restructuring. First Mr E was asked about which skills a package deliverer must have. He mentioned skills like being on time, being friendly, solving problems and availability. Then he was asked to name his best and worst colleague. We finally compared them on the skills he mentioned before. Mr E had to conclude that his skills were almost at the level of his best colleague, and his worrying decreased. Finally, we conducted behavioural experiments where Mr E had to walk through the shopping centre. Here he was prepared in advance by having things to say and having his previously rehearsed attention control strategy. This experience provided a further basis for holding a different and more confident view of himself in the world, so he was able to reduce avoidance and reengage with activities. At the end of the treatment, Mr E was able to resume his job as package deliverer, and improvement on outcome measures was observed.

Case 2: CBT formulation of aggression post-TBI

Robert, a 48-year-old married man with two adult daughters, began a programme of intensive holistic neuropsychological rehabilitation (see Wilson, Gracey, Malley, Bateman, & Evans, 2009) two years after he had sustained severe frontal lobe damage a in a fall during the course of his work on a construction site. As a consequence of the TBI, he exhibited striking impairments of executive function including disinhibition, mental inflexibility, poor self-monitoring and an inability to act on his intentions. As part of this dysexecutive syndrome, he also had severe anger outbursts that threatened his ability to remain in the family home.

In previous rehabilitation, environmental approaches to limit the consequences of Robert's aggression had not been entirely effective, impacting negatively on his mood and self-identity, as he increasingly felt isolated from his family, hopeless about the future, weak and 'useless'. During the holistic programme, Robert worked with a team of rehabilitation staff and his family members to understand the consequences of his injury, set functionally relevant goals for work and family life and attempt to learn to manage his aggression and reduce outbursts whilst increasing his engagement in activities that were meaningful to him.

A longitudinal CBT formulation was developed to help Robert make sense of his aggressive behaviour and to help his family and the other professionals involved in his care to understand. The formulation can be seen in Figure 1.4. This formulation included the initial development of aggression as a behavioural response to negative emotions and experiences during childhood, the beliefs and rules developed at that time and over earlier adult life and the triggers for his aggressive behaviour in the present day.

There was a wide range of specific trigger situations initially. It was necessary to focus on a smaller number of key trigger situations for therapy and rehabilitation, and to understand the core meanings or assumptions associated with triggers. These were situations in which he was unable to complete a task to his own expectations, where others commented or 'interfered' with doing a task, or where he saw other people behaving in ways he disliked (e.g., making errors when driving, as he had not been able to return to driving and thought that this was an injustice). The failure to perform according to his own expectations (as either noticed by himself, or by others) violated rules for living he developed in childhood to feel 'ok' and safe (being emotionally strong, competent, hardworking, being 'the boss' and exerting power over others). The immediate threat response of aggression ('fight') arose in the context of a deeper sense of shame

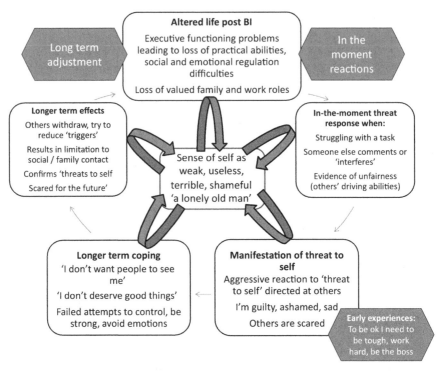

Altered life post BI

Executive functioning problems leading to loss of practical abilities, social and emotional regulation difficulties

Loss of valued family and work roles

Long term adjustment

In the moment reactions

Longer term effects

Others withdraw, try to reduce 'triggers'

Results in limitation to social / family contact

Confirms 'threats to self

Scared for the future'

In-the-moment threat response when:

Struggling with a task

Someone else comments or 'interferes'

Evidence of unfairness (others' driving abilities)

Sense of self as weak, useless, terrible, shameful 'a lonely old man'

Longer term coping

'I don't want people to see me'

'I don't deserve good things'

Failed attempts to control, be strong, avoid emotions

Manifestation of threat to self

Aggressive reaction to 'threat to self' directed at others

I'm guilty, ashamed, sad

Others are scared

Early experiences: To be ok I need to be tough, work hard, be the boss

FIGURE 1.4 Vicious daisy formulation of Robert's 'anger' as arising from a combination of pre-injury experiences, negative core sense of self and failure of pre-injury coping strategies to be effective in managing underlying negative sense of self

and weakness about himself. Although rooted in pre-injury experiences, the difficulties with executive and self-regulatory abilities reduced his ability to manage the trigger (e.g., a set-back or challenge when completing a task) and impacted on relationships and regulation of the negative emotional response itself.

Over time, Robert felt increasingly low, guilty and ashamed, seeing himself as 'terrible'. Coping with this involved either wanting to withdraw or avoid challenges, and he had a period in the past of feeling suicidal. Compounding this, others had previously attempted to help by reducing exposure to triggers, in effect limiting his access to certain people, environments and activities. The formulation of the nature of the underlying threat highlights how this may have had detrimental effects, confirming his unworthiness.

Work with Robert involved developing the formulation with him and sharing it with his family. He was introduced to self-regulatory strategies but found these difficult to implement given his executive difficulties. Formulating and highlighting the underlying reasons for Robert's reactions helped those around him to understand why he was acting the way he did, to re-access their feelings of compassion for him and gain a new perspective on his triggers. In turn this helped to limit Robert's experience of threat and shame as those around him communicated differently and in a way that reinforced Robert's sense of being a person who is loved, valued and worthwhile.

The family was supported to implement a behavioural strategy of helping Robert deescalate situations in which he was triggered. This involved agreeing with his family to postpone the discussion of contentious issues temporarily and using a catchphrase and visual metaphor to support the implementation of this strategy. This collaborative approach supported a sense of agency for Robert, whilst allowing family relationships to improve. The improvement in Robert's aggression is displayed in Figure 1.5. During the rehabilitation programme, in the later phase when reengaging with return to work, 'threats to self' were triggered from a meeting which was intended as helpful, covering a graded return and possibly changing his role.

After the meeting incidents reduced again. Follow up with Robert showed how he used experiences following his intensive rehabilitation to update his sense of identity. He worked in volunteer positions, which allowed him to come to a different understanding of his abilities and seemed to provide a basis for exploring a 'new me'. He also became more realistic about the demands of work by learning from other clients who were struggling with work that was too demanding for them. Robert updated his key priorities from striving to prove himself through achievement to a focus on staying well, having positive interactions with his family and finding enjoyable work that fits with his current interests and abilities. This helped him develop an updated view of himself as someone who can still contribute to his family life whilst recognising his limitations.

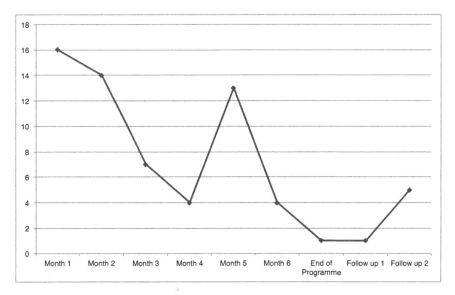

FIGURE 1.5 Number of aggressive episodes as reported by Robert's family using ABC charts over the course of his rehabilitation programme and subsequent follow up

Reflections and discussion

In this chapter we have set out our argument for a cognitive behavioural therapeutic approach with people with ABI, which shares many commonalities with the wider world of CBT practice. However, the approach we propose is uniquely tailored to common challenges faced by people post-injury. The model includes a focus on subjective experience in the moment, subtle variations in emotional (physiological, cognitive, behavioural) changes in day-to-day life and the effects of longer-term coping. However, intervention choice will vary depending on the specific processes involved and specific meanings and coping responses of an individual client. Some in the wider world of CBT currently seem intent on salami-slicing and distinguishing the various CBT 'products' available into behavioural, cognitive, third wave, etc., focusing on differences (perhaps echoing the broader global zeitgeist of neoliberal commodification of human experience and populism) more than commonalities. In our work with people with ABI we must put aside these perceived differences and distinctions, and engage with the creative endeavours at the heart of CBT: the collaborative process of intervention development with others; curiosity and openness to what works rather than what is conceptually 'pure' in that specific school of 'CBT'; and the iterative development of models that guide therapist understanding and build bridges with people who otherwise feel disconnected from themselves and others. It is this humanising and constructive endeavour, bringing with it the potential for emancipation and reduction of suffering and the openness that the CBT community has to diversification and reinvention, which inspires our continued interest and work in this field.

References

Arundine, A., Bradbury, C. L., Dupuis, K., Dawson, D. R., Ruttan, L. A., & Green, R. E. A. (2012). Cognitive behavior therapy after acquired brain injury: Maintenance of therapeutic benefits at 6 months posttreatment. *The Journal of Head Trauma Rehabilitation, 27*(2), 104–112. https://doi.org/10.1097/HTR.0b013e3182125591. Retrieved from http://journals.lww.com/headtraumarehab/Fulltext/2012/03000/Cognitive_Behavior_Therapy_After_Acquired_Brain.4.aspx

Baylan, S., Swann-Price, R., Peryer, G., & Quinn, T. (2016). The effects of music listening interventions on cognition and mood post-stroke: A systematic review. *Expert Review of Neurotherapeutics, 16*(11), 1241–1249. http://doi.org/10.1080/14737175.2016.1227241

Beck, A. T., Rush, A. J., Shaw, B. F., & Emery, G. (1979). *Cognitive therapy of depression.* New York: Guilford Press.

Bédard, M., Felteau, M., Marshall, S., Cullen, N., Gibbons, C., Dubois, S. . . . Moustgaard, A. (2014). Mindfulness-based cognitive therapy reduces symptoms of depression in people with a traumatic brain injury: Results from a randomized controlled trial. *The Journal of Head Trauma Rehabilitation, 29*(4), E13–E22. Retrieved from http://search.ebscohost.com/login.aspx?direct=true&db=psyh&AN=2014-28408-012&site=ehost-live

Bradbury, C. L., Christensen, B. K., Lau, M. A., Ruttan, L. A., Arundine, A. L., & Green, R. E. (2008). The efficacy of cognitive behavior therapy in the treatment of emotional distress after acquired brain injury. *Archives of Physical Medicine and Rehabilitation, 89*(12), S61–S68. https://doi.org/10.1016/j.apmr.2008.08.210

Brindley, R., Bateman, A., & Gracey, F. (2011). Exploration of use of SenseCam to support autobiographical memory retrieval within a cognitive-behavioural therapeutic intervention following acquired brain injury. *Memory, 19*(7), 745–757. https://doi.org/10.1080/09658211.2010.493893

Clark, D. M. (2011). Implementing NICE guidelines for the psychological treatment of depression and anxiety disorders: The IAPT experience. *International Review of Psychiatry, 23*(11), 318–327. http://doi.org/10.3109/09540261.2011.606803

Clark, D. M., & Wells, A. (1995). A cognitive model of social phobia. In R. G. Heimberg, M. R. Liebowitz, D. A. Hope, & F. R. Schneier (Eds.), *Social phobia: Diagnosis, assessment and treatment*. New York: Guilford Press.

Corrie, S., & Lane, D. (2015). *CBT supervision*. London: Sage Publications.

Cullen, B., Pownall, J., Cummings, J., Baylan, S., Broomfield, N., Haig, C. . . . Evans, J. J. (2018). Positive PsychoTherapy in ABI Rehab (PoPsTAR): A pilot randomised controlled trial. *Neuropsychological Rehabilitation, 28*(1), 17–33. http://doi.org/10.1080/09602011.2015.1131722

Dewar, B.-K., & Gracey, F. (2007). "Am not was": Cognitive-behavioural therapy for adjustment and identity change following herpes simplex encephalitis. *Neuropsychological Rehabilitation, 17*(4–5). http://doi.org/10.1080/09602010601051610

Ellis-Hill, C., Gracey, F., Thomas, S., Lamont-Robinson, C., Thomas, P. W., Marques, E. M. R. . . . Jenkinson, D. F. (2015). "HeART of Stroke (HoS)", a community-based arts for health group intervention to support self-confidence and psychological well-being following a stroke: Protocol for a randomised controlled feasibility study. *BMJ Open, 5*(8). http://doi.org/10.1136/bmjopen-2015-008888

Gallagher, M., McLeod, H. J., & McMillan, T. M. (2019). A systematic review of recommended modifications of CBT for people with cognitive impairments following brain injury. *Neuropsychological Rehabilitation, 29*(1), 1–21. http://doi.org/10.1080/09602011.2016.1258367

Galvin, K. T., & Todres, L. (2011). Kinds of well-being: A conceptual framework that provides direction for caring. *International Journal of Qualitative Studies on Health and Well-being, 6*(4). http://doi.org/10.3402/qhw.v6i4.10362

Gertler, P., Tate, R. L., & Cameron, I. D. (2015). Non-pharmacological interventions for depression in adults and children with traumatic brain injury. *Cochrane Database of Systematic Reviews, 12*, CD009871. https://doi.org/10.1002/14651858.CD009871.pub2

Goldstein, K. (1952). The effect of brain damage on the personality. *Psychiatry: Journal for the Study of Interpersonal Processes, 15*(3), 245–260.

Gracey, F., Brentnall, S., & Megoran, R. (2009). Judith: Learning to do things "at the drop of a hat": Behavioural experiments to explore and change the "meaning" in meaningful functional activity. In B. Wilson, F. Gracey, J. Evans, & A. Bateman (Eds.), *Neuropsychological rehabilitation: Theory, models, therapy and outcome* (pp. 256–271). Cambridge: Cambridge University Press. http://doi.org/10.1017/CBO9780511581083.019

Gracey, F., Evans, J. J., & Malley, D. (2009). Capturing process and outcome in complex rehabilitation interventions: A "Y-shaped" model. *Neuropsychological Rehabilitation, 19*(6), 867–890. http://doi.org/10.1080/09602010903027763

Gracey, F., Ford, C., & Psaila, K. (2015). A provisional transdiagnostic cognitive behavioural model of post brain injury emotional adjustment. *Neuro-Disability and Psychotherapy, 3*(3), 154–185.

Gracey, F., Malley, D., & Evans, J. J. (2009). Interdisciplinary vocational rehabilitation addressing pain, fatigue, anxiety and impulsivity: Yusuf and his "new rules for business and life". In B. Wilson, F. Gracey, J. Evans, & A. Bateman (Eds.), *Neuropsychological rehabilitation: Theory, models, therapy and outcome*. Cambridge: Cambridge University Press. http://doi.org/10.1017/CBO9780511581083.018

Gracey, F., Oldham, P., & Kritzinger, R. (2007). Finding out if "the 'me' will shut down": Successful cognitive-behavioural therapy of seizure-related panic symptoms following subarachnoid haemorrhage: A single case report. *Neuropsychological Rehabilitation, 17*(1). http://doi.org/10.1080/09602010500505260

Gracey, F., Prince, L., & Winson, R. (2017). Working with identity change after brain injury. In R. Winson, B. A. Wilson, & A. Bateman (Eds.), *The brain injury rehabilitation workbook*. New York: Guilford Press.

Hackett, M., Anderson, C., House, A., & Halteh, C. (2008). Interventions for preventing depression after stroke. *Cochrane Database of Systematic Reviews, 3*. http://doi.org/10.1002/14651858.CD003689.pub3

Hsieh, M. Y., Ponsford, J., Wong, D., Schönberger, M., Taffe, J., & McKay, A. (2012). Motivational interviewing and cognitive behaviour therapy for anxiety following traumatic brain injury: A pilot randomised controlled trial. *Neuropsychological Rehabilitation, 22*(4), 585–608.

Judd, D., & Wilson, S. L. (2005). Psychotherapy with brain injury survivors: An investigation of the challenges encountered by clinicians and their modifications to therapeutic practice. *Brain Injury, 19*(6), 437–449. http://doi.org/10.1080/02699050400010994

King, N., Pimm, J., & Tyerman, A. (2014). Enhancing the integration of psychological services for stroke patients through the development of a protocol for neuropsychology and IAPT services. *Clinical Psychology Forum, 255*(March), 19–21.

Kneebone, I. (2015). Stepped psychological care after stroke. *Disability and Rehabilitation, 38*(18), 1836–1843. http://doi.org/10.3109/09638288.2015.1107764

LeDoux, J. (2003). The emotional brain, fear, and the amygdala. *Cellular and Molecular Neurobiology, 23*(4–5), 727–738.

Mansell, W., Harvey, A., Watkins, E. R., & Shafran, R. (2008). Cognitive behavioral processes across psychological disorders: A review of the utility and validity of the transdiagnostic approach. *International Journal of Cognitive Therapy, 1*(3), 181–191. http://doi.org/10.1680/ijct.2008.1.3.181

McGrath, J., King, N., Bennett-Levy, J., Butler, G., Fennell, M., Hackman, A. . . . Westbrook, D. (2004). *Oxford guide to behavioural experiments in cognitive therapy*. Oxford: Oxford University Press.

Mooney, K. A., & Padesky, C. A. (2000). Applying client creativity to recurrent problems: Constructing possibilities and tolerating doubt. *Journal of Cognitive Psychotherapy, 14*(2), 149–161.

National Collaborating Centre for Mental Health. (2018). *The IAPT pathway for people with long-term physical health conditions and medically unexplained symptoms*. London: National Collaborating Centre for Mental Health. Retrieved from https://www.rcpsych.ac.uk/docs/default-source/improving-care/nccmh/nccmh-iapt-ltc-full-implementation-guidance.pdf?sfvrsn=de824ea4_4

National Institute for Health and Clinical Evidence. (2011). *Common mental health problems: Identification and pathways to care*. NICE Clinical Guideline [CG123]. Retrieved January 25, 2019 from www.nice.org.uk/guidance/cg123

Ownsworth, T., Fleming, J., Strong, J., Radel, M., Chan, W., & Clare, L. (2007). Awareness typologies, long-term emotional adjustment and psychosocial outcomes following acquired brain injury. *Neuropsychological Rehabilitation, 17*(2), 129–150.

Ownsworth, T., Gooding, K., & Beadle, E. (2019). Self-focused processing after severe traumatic brain injury: Relationship to neurocognitive functioning and mood symptoms. *British Journal of Clinical Psychology, 58*(1), 35–50. http://doi.org/10.1111/bjc.12185

Ownsworth, T., & Gracey, F. (2017). Cognitive behavioural therapy for people with brain injury. In B. A. Wilson, J. Winegardner, C. M. van Heugten, & T. Ownsworth (Eds.), *Neuropsychological rehabilitation: The international handbook*. London: Routledge.

Ownsworth, T., & Haslam, C. (2016). Impact of rehabilitation on self-concept following traumatic brain injury: An exploratory systematic review of intervention methodology and efficacy. *Neuropsychological Rehabilitation, 26*(1), 1–35. http://doi.org/10.1080/09602011.2014.977924

Powell, T., Ekin-Wood, A., & Collin, C. (2007). Post-traumatic growth after head injury: A long-term follow-up. *Brain Injury, 21*(1), 31–38.

Schmidt, J., Fleming, J., Ownsworth, T., & Lannin, N. A. (2013). Video feedback on functional task performance improves self-awareness after traumatic brain injury: A randomized controlled trial. *Neurorehabilitation and Neural Repair, 27*(4), 316–324. http://doi.org/10.1177/1545968312469838

Schmidt, J., Lannin, N., Fleming, J., & Ownsworth, T. (2011). Feedback interventions for impaired self-awareness following brain injury: A systematic review. *Journal of Rehabilitation Medicine, 43*(8), 673–680. http://doi.org/10.2340/16501977-0846

Shields, C., Ownsworth, T., O'Donovan, A., & Fleming, J. (2016). A transdiagnostic investigation of emotional distress after traumatic brain injury. *Neuropsychological Rehabilitation, 26*(3), 410–445. http://doi.org/10.1080/09602011.2015.1037772

Silva, J., Ownsworth, T., Shields, C., & Fleming, J. (2011). Enhanced appreciation of life following acquired brain injury: Posttraumatic growth at 6 months postdischarge. *Brain Impairment, 12*(2), 93–104.

Simblett, S. K., Yates, M., Wagner, A. P., Watson, P., Gracey, F., Ring, H., & Bateman, A. (2017). Computerized cognitive behavioral therapy to treat emotional distress after stroke: A feasibility randomized controlled trial. *JMIR Mental Health, 4*(2), e16. http://doi.org/10.2196/mental.6022

Simpson, G. K., Tate, R. L., Whiting, D. L., & Cotter, R. E. (2011). Suicide prevention after traumatic brain injury: A randomized controlled trial of a program for the psychological treatment of hopelessness. *Journal of Head Trauma Rehabilitation, 26*(4), 290–300.

Soo, C., & Tate, R. (2007). Psychological treatment for anxiety in people with traumatic brain injury. *Cochrane Database of Systematic Reviews, 3*, CD005239. http://doi.org/10.1002/14651858.CD005239.pub2

Stalder-Lüthy, F., Messerli-Bürgy, N., Hofer, H., Frischknecht, E., Znoj, H., & Barth, J. (2013). Effect of psychological interventions on depressive symptoms in long-term rehabilitation after an acquired brain injury: A systematic review and meta-analysis. *Archives of Physical Medicine and Rehabilitation, 94*(7), 1386–1397. https://doi.org/10.1016/j.apmr.2013.02.013

Teasdale, J. D., & Barnard, P. J. (1993). *Affect, cognition and change: Remodelling depressive thought*. London: Lawrence Erlbaum Associates.

Tedeschi, R. G., & Calhoun, L. G. (2004). Posttraumatic growth: Conceptual foundations and empirical evidence. *Psychological Inquiry, 15*(1), 1–18. http://doi.org/10.1207/s15327965pli1501_01

Thomas, S. A., Walker, M. F., MacNiven, J. A., Haworth, H., & Lincoln, N. B. (2013). Communication and Low Mood (CALM): A randomized controlled trial of behavioural therapy for stroke patients with aphasia. *Clinical Rehabilitation, 27*(5), 398–408. http://doi.org/10.1177/0269215512462227

Waldron, B., Casserly, L. M., & O'Sullivan, C. (2013). Cognitive behavioural therapy for depression and anxiety in adults with acquired brain injury. What works for whom? *Neuropsychological Rehabilitation, 23*(1), 64–101.

Wells, A. (1997). *Cognitive therapy of anxiety disorders: A practical guide.* Chichester: Wiley-Blackwell.

Wilson, B. A., Gracey, F., Malley, D., Bateman, A., & Evans, J. J. (2009). The Oliver Zangwill Centre approach to neuropsychological rehabilitation. In B. Wilson, F. Gracey, J. Evans, & A. Bateman (Eds.), *Neuropsychological rehabilitation: Theory, models, therapy and outcome* (pp. 47–67). Cambridge: Cambridge University Press.

Yeates, G., Henwood, K., Gracey, F., & Evans, J. (2007). Awareness of disability after acquired brain injury and the family context. *Neuropsychological Rehabilitation, 17*(2), 151–173. http://doi.org/777126249[pii]10.1080/09602010600696423

2

ACCEPTANCE AND COMMITMENT THERAPY (ACT) AFTER BRAIN INJURY

David Todd and Mike Smith

Acceptance and Commitment Therapy (ACT) is a third-wave cognitive behavioural therapy that is rooted in both pragmatic philosophical traditions and radical behaviourism. A large body of empirical research has been undertaken over the last 30 years that supports Relational Frame Theory (RFT – which emerged from radical behaviourism), the theory that underpins ACT. Consideration of RFT is beyond the scope of this chapter, but interested readers are encouraged to consult Törneke (2010). During the last 15 years ACT has been used increasingly in populations with neurological conditions, including traumatic brain injury (e.g., Myles, 2004; Whiting, Deane, Simpson, McLeod, & Ciarrochi, 2017).

Theoretical and philosophical basis of the therapy

ACT views language as the ultimate source of clinical problems. Complex language is unique to the human race and coincidentally so is suffering in the absence of any proximal cause. Some theorists have suggested that this is in part because language has evolved in a spectacularly successful fashion to aid our survival as a species (e.g., Pinker, 1997), and therefore is problem-focused. Language, and the benefit it confers in being able to describe the world and communicate those descriptions, has made us quite literally the masters of our universe. We have an extraordinary level of control over our environment relative to our pre language ancestors or animals that do not use complex abstract language.

Language describes the world as a collection of things (e.g., people, fish, oceans, cars), and names them as such. Language can also provide a description of how those things interact or fit together (e.g., people drive cars, fish swim in oceans). Language therefore is really good at making the world seem like a great big machine the parts of which fit together and 'work' together to 'give' us our world. The logical extension is that the whole world is knowable if we can figure out how all the parts fit together.

ACT sees the world in a different way. Whilst language is still seen as being a system of symbols that relate to real world 'things', it is the context in which things are contained (and critically the associated action) that is of more interest. Furthermore, the things and the action are only considered in respect of the outcome that is desired in context. For example, we can readily consider the various forms that a song comes in. A song can be recorded on an MP3 player, it can be played on a guitar, it can be written down as a musical score. What we want to do with the song governs which is most useful. We couldn't play the music score in our car, the MP3 player would be better, and we couldn't readily use the MP3 player as a musical instrument at a live performance. Critically then the context governs which format of the same song is most useful or 'works'. In thinking of 'worlds', this is particularly true of our internal world. Whilst we have amazing technology at our disposal for changing or controlling the physical world (buildings shelter us from weather, sea defences stop flooding, drugs fight infections), the same control and change approach is not so readily useful for the content of our minds.

While this might seem an academic distinction, it actually has great implications for practice. If we approach a problem with the aim of doing what works, we can avoid getting into arguments with clients about who or what is right (or how much of the immediate therapy 'world' under consideration we can know and agree on). There are then a different set of assumptions that underpin ACT relative to other forms of psychotherapy, most of which are likely to be founded on a structural and mechanistic way of viewing the world that language provides so readily. For example, most therapists would have no problem with, and indeed would readily add into a formulation, the statement, 'I can't go to my friend's wedding because I'm anxious that I'll have a panic attack'. The situation posed in that statement is also enshrined in the DSM-V criteria for agoraphobia (APA, 2013). The philosophical underpinnings of ACT would view that statement as not necessarily true but rather more worthy of functional analysis. For example, what does disclosing that statement elicit from others? What contexts has that not happened in? What imagined and similar context would there be less anxiety associated with? Is there really a causal link present (going to wedding = panic attack)? Thus it can be seen that thoughts in many psychotherapies are viewed as independent variables, they *cause* the unhelpful behaviour. The ACT practitioner would see thoughts, feelings and behaviours as dependent variables, that is they are consequential to a particular context, and it is the context that allows for manipulation and change (and therefore is the independent variable). The target is therefore the arbitrary associations between aversive psychological experiences, rather than the psychological experiences themselves.

Great emphasis in the ACT model is placed on workability: avoiding being right and focusing on what works is liberating and provides clinical focus without being side-tracked by an absolute desire to be right. The desire to be right is sourced in forms of rule-following that are unique to humans, but not exhibited in animals (the term 'rule-governed' behaviour is used in ACT when responses are controlled by a verbal description of a contingency rather than the contingency itself). For example, if a rat is put into a maze and is allowed to search for food hidden in the maze it will, through exploration, eventually find the food. If this is repeated multiple times, the rat will learn the fastest route to get to the food with relative ease. If however, when this is a well-established behaviour, the rat is put into a maze and there is no food in the location it was originally, the rat will sniff and search for a while before moving on to see if there is food located somewhere else. What the rat won't do is sit down at the spot and exclaim that it just isn't fair as food has always been there before, and so should be there now. This is exactly what most humans do on a daily basis. Think of how irritated and 'stuck' on the unfairness of a situation people may become if for example a road is unexpectedly closed on their route to work, and the detour makes them late. It is likely that the first utterance to colleagues will be about how unreasonable or unfair it was.

In ACT sessions, techniques are developed in order to undermine unworkable rules and promote adaptive rules ('rules' and 'language' are interchangeable here). This requires a 'new mode of mind' and is not therefore just a technique that can be readily stuffed into a clinical bag of tricks. ACT is based on an 'assumption of destructive normality', promoting a mindfulness and acceptance-based approach entailing a willingness to experience odd or uncomfortable thoughts, feelings, or physical sensations in order to respond with 'psychological flexibility'. Psychological flexibility is defined as the ability to connect with the present moment and experience the thoughts and feelings without unhelpful defence, and to persist in action that is consistent with values, or change that action when the situation demands (Kim et al., 2011). ACT assumes that suffering is a normal and an unavoidable part of human experience, and our very attempts to control or avoid painful experiences in fact contribute to long-term suffering (e.g., Harris, 2007). Minds are therefore seen as not having evolved to make us feel happy, but to keep us alive. ACT differs from therapeutic models which prioritise symptom reduction (such as CBT), as psychological flexibility does not directly aim to change 'happiness' or 'freedom from pain', which ACT explains are counterproductive targets for pursuit.

ACT uses a 'hexaflex' model (Hayes, Luoma, Bond, Masuda, & Lillis, 2006; see Figure 2.1) with which to explore progress on the different interacting six core processes of psychological flexibility (for an accessible introduction to the ACT model see Harris & Hayes, 2009). These different processes are used in therapy to chart progress in skill acquisition to bolster psychological flexibility. Increases in these skills of psychological flexibility outlined in the Hexaflex enable progress to be made with difficulties such as 'cognitive fusion', 'experiential avoidance', 'unworkable action' and 'struggle with feelings' rooted in unworkable 'rules' that are, in fact, arbitrary associations (i.e., our minds might try to convince us they are factual or 'true' but they most certainly may not be).

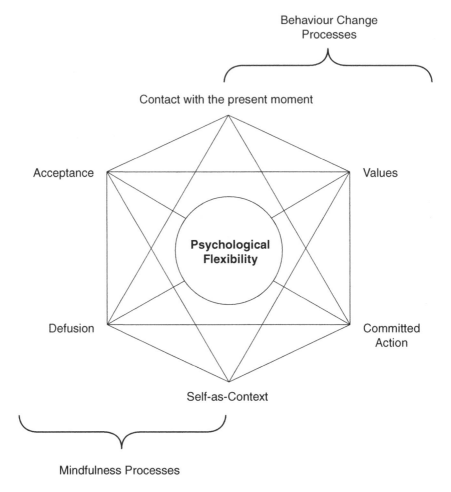

FIGURE 2.1   ACT 'Hexaflex' (Hayes et al., 2006)

Core elements of ACT model (as outlined in the Hexaflex)

The six core therapeutic processes that configure the Hexaflex are: contact with the present moment, self-as-context, acceptance, cognitive defusion, values and committed action (Hayes et al., 2003). The therapist can elect to work on any of the components of this interactive and nonlinear model at any stage of the therapy process, or these components can be combined and presented at the same time, for example:

 Be Present – 'You are here and now' ('contact with the present moment' and 'self-as-context'): The focus of *contact with the present moment* is consciously connecting with what is happening in that moment, including practicing mindfulness and metacognitive skills. These skills support us to develop *self-as-context* (or the observing self), recognising that a component of us is always the same, rather than 'self-as-content', which involves fusing with unhelpful labels about the self. This approach can be useful in reframing the associations of loss and deficit, common after acquired brain injury, and supporting the process of acceptance, adjustment and adaptation. These ACT processes are aiming to facilitate a process of detachment from the unhelpful content of our lives and realising that associations with the past and future 'exist' only in the present. Reasoning and evaluating evidence may be particularly difficult when the person is cognitively impaired; however, addressing thoughts such as 'my brain injury stops me doing what I used to do' or 'I'm not the same person as I was before my brain injury' by using an ACT approach reduces this problem of trying to challenge thoughts after brain injury (Whiting, Deane, Simpson, McLeod, & Ciarrochi, 2015).

Open Up – 'You are not your thoughts or feelings . . .' ('acceptance' and 'defusion'): *Acceptance* is making room for distressing thoughts, emotions or experiences so that there is no longer an ongoing struggle, whilst simultaneous *defusion* from unhelpful thoughts refers to the process of creating some separation from these internal experiences. The idea is of neither believing unhelpful thoughts nor trying to suppress them but instead trying to develop a new way of engaging with them. This can be a difficult message to explain verbally. Hence, metaphors and experiential learning are a strong component of an ACT approach (see Appendix 1 – Useful information on ACT resources). The aim is to foster an active choice to use the opportunity to experience emotional discomfort but in an augmented form or through a different lens of perception; A detached interest in one's own private experiences.

Do What Matters – '. . . you are your values, and your actions guided by these values' ('values' and 'committed action'): The focus on doing what matters, identifying *values* that are unique and personally relevant to each individual and *committed action* towards these values represents a concrete and measurable behavioural baseline through goal setting. In addition, the focus on values is useful for moving away from distinctions of pre-injury/post-injury, as personal values typically are continuous and unaffected by brain injury (although of course a person's values may change over time). Identified values provide signposts for rehabilitation goals and enable the person to direct their rehabilitation team. For example, self-as-content may define the person as failing to meet their pre-morbid goals (e.g., being the highest goal-scorer at the football club, getting the promotion at work), however values (and the principles that usually serve the value) provide the higher-order direction of travel to develop goals for committed action (e.g., perseverance towards success, determination and resilience when facing challenges). A number of process measures are available for support in values identification, e.g., The Survey of Life Principles Version 2.2 – Card Sorting Task (CST; Ciarrochi & Bailey, 2008).

Considerations for ACT following brain injury

Cognitive strengths and difficulties (attention, language, memory, executive functioning): A consideration with ACT, and other forms of psychotherapy, when working with people after brain injury is whether the person can engage in talking therapy and remember the content. ACT is a less prescriptive approach relative to other therapies and can be applied flexibly to suit the needs of the individual, with as much structure being implemented as required to meet the cognitive strengths and difficulties of a person following brain injury. Consideration needs to be made as to whether external structure and compensatory strategies need to be implemented to address cognitive barriers. Much of ACT intervention is completed 'in the moment', which negates the 'stuckness' of not having completed homework or other tasks. In addition, ACT seeks to draw on retained memory pathways through experiential therapeutic processes, thus engaging implicit memory resources to support learning. Where cognitive flexibility is impaired, acceptance of unpleasant thoughts can be facilitated by using concrete strategies such as 'physicalising' the thought (Hayes et al., 2003). Another advantage of ACT with people following brain injury is that many resources are available in video and pictorial representations (see Appendix 1); information is therefore delivered in more than one modality in order to support difficulties with processing information (Simpson, Tate, Whiting, & Cotter, 2011). It is further suggested that ACT is well positioned to work with people experiencing cognitive impairment, as the ability to work towards psychological flexibility and persist with values-consistent behaviour, despite acquired impairments, is a key target for intervention following brain injury.

'Cognitive flexibility' versus 'Psychological flexibility': As described, psychological flexibility is proposed to be necessary for wellbeing in ACT, and a component of psychological flexibility is cognitive flexibility, which can be impaired as a result of difficulties with executive processes following brain injury. However, recent research has suggested that people with brain injury often have a positive response to therapies that promote psychological flexibility, despite reduced cognitive flexibility (Whiting, Deane, Simpson, McLeod et al., 2017). Whiting and colleagues found that, overall, psychological flexibility appears a more overarching construct and cognitive flexibility may be a subcomponent of it but not necessarily a pre-requisite. Indeed, in clinical practice the authors (MS and DT) have found that ACT concepts/ strategies themselves are useful in addressing difficulties presented through impaired cognitive flexibility (e.g., concrete thinking, perseveration) through fostering a new relationship with the mind. For example, the therapist helps the client notice and explore direct experience and identify emotion control strategies, and to 'defuse' the client from the mind's content and direct attention to the moment. Consistent with a 'stop and think' approach to cognitive rehabilitation after brain injury, the ACT therapist detects when the client is drifting into the past or future and teaches the client how to come back to the here and now. Whiting et al. (2015) suggest that ACT may benefit people with brain injury by improving both psychological flexibility and cognitive flexibility. However, there is a need for research into cognitive rehabilitation or treatment studies addressing impairments into cognitive flexibility (and other executive functioning) and measures of psychological flexibility.

Insight and acceptance: A barrier to engagement in psychotherapy is often described as the client's impaired level of awareness of their acquired deficits, and their ability to accept and cope realistically with those losses. ACT as an acceptance-based approach aims to support people to develop new skills, rather than focusing on what has been lost (particularly relevant following brain injury). However, knowing the person's progress after injury through the process of awareness, acceptance and adjustment, enables the structure and delivery of the therapy to be guided. The therapeutic stance that everyone has a mind that is often negatively focused (including the therapist) facilitates less of a power imbalance. In addition, the focus of values in ACT is useful for shared goals despite difficulties with insight and awareness ('you can always do something that you value, if you truly value it'). In addition, ACT provides interventions to address challenges in therapy or rehabilitation presented by reduced insight or awareness, including explicitly communicating that the client is simply using unworkable strategies which can be revised. In addition, the therapist actively contrasts what the client's 'mind' says will work versus what the client's experience says is working. If the client is presenting with thoughts such as 'There's nothing wrong with me', and his family are constantly pointing out his cognitive and behavioural deficits, he is likely to become entrenched. Revisiting such a scenario from a being right as opposed to a 'what is working' perspective is what is often incorporated in other forms of psychological work on insight (although not necessarily framed in those terms). ACT would also encourage the person to pay attention to and become less fused with concomitant thoughts such as 'But I am right, there's nothing wrong with me, they don't know what they're talking about', which people lacking insight often have about significant others. Ultimately, the therapist helps the person to elucidate their 'story' whilst highlighting the potentially unworkable results of literal attachment to the story.

Goal setting: The process of goal-setting is the most appropriate way to plan, direct and measure the success of rehabilitation (Wilson, Evans, & Gracey, 2009). ACT can represent an effective approach in teaching clients to distinguish between values and goals, to distinguish between goals (outcomes) and the process of striving toward goals (growth that occurs as a result of striving). However, the ACT therapist accepts the client's values and, if unwilling to work with them, refers the client on to another provider or community resource. In other words, ACT outlines that the therapist helps the client develop their own personal value-based goals and build a concrete action plan around them, including with the wider rehabilitation team. During the process of rehabilitation/ therapy, the ACT approach helps client distinguish between deciding and choosing to engage in committed action and encourages the client to make and keep commitments in the presence of perceived barriers (e.g., fear of failure, plateau in physical recovery from injury). For example, values create an opportunity to define and personalise goals in order to make them more client-focused and relevant to the client. It is the experience of the authors (DT & MS) that this fits well with MDT working in neurorehabilitation and is easily integrated within the context of the wider rehabilitation team.

Values – a compass for adjustment?: Frequently following brain injury, clients can become stuck on how unfair their predicament is and will often make conditional statements (e.g., if I cannot walk again, life is not worth living). The use of values can be a powerful and collaborative way of helping a client adjust to whatever disability and handicap their brain injury related impairment is affecting. The example given earlier is one that I'm sure that most professionals working in neurorehabilitation have encountered. A person has lost or reduced physical ability, and the combined effect of rigidity, egocentricity and reduced impulse control results in the person becoming stuck and making conditional statements. Usually when we walk we do it in the service of doing something else. It is true that we can walk just for the sake of walking, but even that is not an isolated experiential exercise. We could say, 'I really value walking on the moors', but we wouldn't realistically walk with a blindfold and earmuffs on. 'Walking on the moors' also involves appreciating the sights and sounds of the moors so whilst we value the physical act of walking, we are always exposed to other facets of an activity in most things we do. Returning to our brain injury survivor it is true that they might value walking per se, but it is also the case that they value what walking 'gives' us, predominantly independence. Using values then it is productive to explore with the client what walking 'gives' them that they are missing. In doing this ways can be explored to find alternative methods of gaining access to the same valued experience. For example, one client related that he was not interested in rehab if he could not walk. Exploration of his values suggested that this was predominantly because he was an avid golfer premorbidly. Given that he had a dense left hemiplegia, the prospect of him walking or playing golf again was greatly reduced. He stated in the values assessment however that he really missed playing golf. Using a standing wheelchair, short-range clubs and interdisciplinary working with Occupational Therapy, Physiotherapy and Psychology, he was able to participate in 'pitch and putt' golfing activity. This inevitably bought up cognitive evaluations such as, 'If I can't hit a ball 250 metres with a driver, it's not worth playing'. Such evaluations can then be tackled using cognitive defusion, acceptance and self as context techniques, as if the person really values the playing of golf, then playing is what matters.

Similarly, lack of insight can also be usefully helped by the use of a structured values-based approach. Most people who lack insight experience social challenges to a greater or lesser degree. Interpersonal relationships are almost always problematic, and a client's lack of awareness is usually near the top of any problem list a family reports during assessment. Critically the client, usually, values their interpersonal relationships greatly, and the paradox of them 'talking a good game' by saying they love their nearest and dearest, whilst engaging in behaviours that are a product of poor insight can be both frustrating and hurtful for the family. The use of values in conjunction with workability as previously discussed can be a powerful mediator of acceptance and behavioural change. One of us (MS) worked with a stroke survivor who was continually accusing his wife of being unfaithful. This was due to a combination of his cognitive deficits and historical factors pertaining to his first marriage. The accusations were causing his wife a considerable amount of distress given that they had been happily married for the preceding 40 years. Each time she was accused by her husband of some implausible act of infidelity (such as taking a bath with a male staff nurse on the ward), she became extremely distressed. Using values in a structured way, we identified why he valued his wife and what the relationship meant to him, particularly given his altered sense of self post-stroke. This work highlighted his wife's unconditional acceptance of the situation and the love she felt for him. We also explored how workable it was to keep making accusations when he knew that they were very upsetting for his wife. His mind on the one hand generating accusations, and then subsequently generating guilt cognitions when he realised they were aberrant thoughts rather than facts. Encouraging him to commit to loving and caring behaviours in the face of such thoughts rapidly reduced the frequency of his accusations (but tellingly the frequency of the thoughts did not reduce over the therapy period).

Suitability: Given that psychological flexibility requires attendance to factors that influence behaviour, as well as being able to inhibit undesired behaviour, there has been concern raised that impaired cognitive flexibility after brain injury will not be able to engage in ACT. However, support for ACT after brain injury has been explored in two recent reviews (Kangas & McDonald, 2011; Soo, Tate, & Lane-Brown, 2011). Much of the available evidence has focused on mild to moderate acquired brain injury, however there is emerging evidence that ACT can be successfully applied even following 'severe' traumatic brain injury (e.g., Whiting et al., 2015). The multimodal approach allows the therapist to make modifications to account for individual differences in cognitive impairment. The process of cognitive defusion removes the need for intellectualising and reasoning. In addition, Whiting, Deane, Simpson, McLeod, & Ciarrochi, (2017) outline therapy modifications to account for cognitive impairments, in terms of both general strategies for CBT and ACT and ACT-specific strategies (see Appendix 2 – Suggested therapy modifications). Due to the need to compensate for differing cognitive impairments it has been proposed that ACT is best delivered individually after brain injury. However, previous interventions after brain injury have been provided in a small group format (e.g., Anson & Ponsford, 2006), and a recent study suggests that ACT can be delivered in a dyad after severe TBI, in order to incorporate some elements of group process but allow for individualisation of therapy (Whiting, Deane, Simpson, Ciarrochi, & McLeod, 2017).

Clinical reflections

In reflecting as regular practitioners of ACT with people after brain injury, the authors (MS and DT) offer our personal reflections on the application of this therapeutic approach with people following brain injury. An important consideration in this context is how an ACT approach sits with the role of being an 'expert' in neuropsychological rehabilitation, for example, 'creative hopelessness' involves acknowledgement that we, as experts, cannot 'fix' the brain injury (as part of promoting willing acceptance of psychological discomfort). In addition, some practitioners may feel uneasy with the dismantling of the traditional power structures inherent in therapist-client relationship, including appropriate use of self-disclosure by the clinician (for example to demonstrate the 'assumption of destructive normality' it is normal to have negative thoughts). However, we have found that the ACT approach is useful in negotiating the dialectic between hope and acceptance, i.e., compensating for acquired impairments after brain injury whilst willingly accepting uncomfortable thoughts and feelings ('Freedom is the knowledge of what is and what isn't in our power to control', Seneca, 49AD).

The ACT focus of skill development (the six core processes of psychological flexibility outlined in the Hexaflex) is consistent with positive psychology principles and developing a skill set, which represents a good fit with neuropsychological rehabilitation, e.g., the development of client-centred goals. In addition, the acceptance-based aspect of ACT is readily applied following the often life-changing trauma and loss associated with brain injury. ACT is compatible with elements of cognitive behavioural therapy (CBT), and physical relaxation interventions, used in other behavioural therapies, are also compatible with meta-cognitive interventions incorporated in cognitive rehabilitation, e.g., attention training/mindfulness.

In addition, ACT resources are freely available on the internet, including in engaging younger demographic disproportionally affected by brain injury, such as YouTube videos for ACT therapeutic metaphors (see Appendix 1). Our experience is that the use of metaphors to communicate to people with brain injury can be a creative opportunity to concretely communicate an understanding of the individual's emotions by the clinician and to strengthen the therapeutic relationship. In addition, it has been noted that clinically it appears that people often seem to find it easier to remember the content of sessions through the use of metaphors presented by the therapist (e.g., Ylvisaker, McPherson, Kayes, & Pellett, 2008).

Following brain injury, difficulties with attention and executive functioning may present, which could provide challenges for psychotherapeutic intervention. We would argue that the focus of ACT of attendance on thoughts, feelings and the contexts in which behaviour takes place, and the aim to inhibit undesired behaviour, is not a reason to exclude those following a brain injury, but, in fact, difficulties suggesting an ACT approach may be indicated.

Case study

A recent case example is described here based on work of one of the authors (DT) in order to exemplify some of the processes in assessment, formulation and intervention based on an ACT approach after brain injury.

Background

On an October evening, Aaron, 22 years old, had been on a night out in town and was being driven home with a group of friends, the car lost control and drove into a lamp-post. Aaron suffered a number of injuries, including a left subdural hematoma, left temporal and bi-frontal contusions; he required a decompressive craniotomy, a neurosurgical procedure to control brain swelling, in order to save his life. His next memory was of living in a neurorehabilitation unit approximately three months later (indicating a severe traumatic brain injury), after intensive treatment, he was eventually discharged home about ten months after the collision. In addition to physical pain and headaches, Aaron had a number of differences in his cognitive, emotional, behavioural and relational functioning. Although cognitive testing indicated that his intellectual functioning was in the 'average' range, he had memory difficulties and significant problems with executive functioning, including planning and organising his thinking and actions; Aaron was described as experiencing 'dysexecutive syndrome' (and therefore would meet the definition of impaired 'cognitive flexibility').

Assessment and referral

Aaron was referred to our service for further neuropsychological intervention approximately five years after receiving his injuries, at 27 years old. At this time, he was living independently in a rented flat in the city centre, and he received rehabilitation support from an interdisciplinary team, including provision of support workers within his home during weekdays. At the time of referral he had suspended his placement on a university course studying media; he had initially asked to manage on his course without support but was struggling. Feedback from his coursework (typically submitted late) was that the essays contained good information, but they were chaotic and disorganised. He struggled to attend teaching sessions and divide attention to take notes during lectures. This course represented his second attempt at higher education following TBI, having dropped out of college two years previously. Aaron presented with low self-esteem; he described loneliness and frustration (Figure 2.2).

Intervention

The aim of ACT intervention was to work with Aaron in the context of a multidisciplinary rehabilitation team approach addressing his person-centred rehabilitation goals. Twelve clinical neuropsychology treatment sessions, 60 minutes in duration, were facilitated on a weekly or fortnightly basis. The principle approach was to apply a framework of ACT, accommodating for neuropsychological strengths and difficulties, in order to reduce struggle against, or fusion with, unhelpful thoughts and feelings, and to increase engagement in actions reflecting his identified personal values. Interdisciplinary work with occupational therapy and with support worker was also indicated in order to support behavioural activation in functional tasks:

- Initial sessions focused on use of **'creative hopelessness'**; Exercises completed to explore whether it was possible or not to control the mind (used

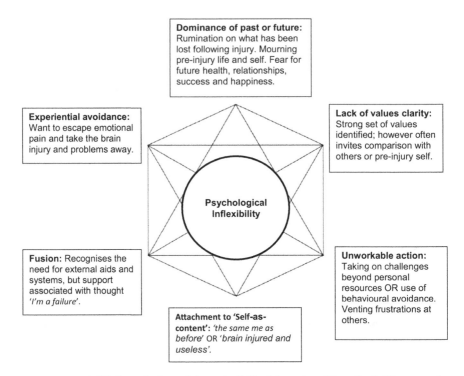

FIGURE 2.2 ACT formulation of Aaron's difficulties using 'Hexaflex' (Hayes et al., 2006)

Source: Copyright Steven C. Hayes. Used by permission

'chocolate cake' exercise). Information provided on the evolutionary context for the functioning of the human mind. Aaron agreed to continue on the premise that trying to escape emotional pain will never work and those attempts to control the mind is the problem (discussed the difference between 'experiential avoidance'/'cognitive fusion' versus 'willingness').

- Focused on supporting Aaron to 'open up' and willingly accept uncomfortable private experiences – Aaron demonstrated good ability to distinguish between situations, thoughts, feelings, and actions. Reinforced that the aim is not to try to eliminate thoughts or feelings, but instead changing the relatedness of certain private experiences (used 'passengers on a bus' and 'unwanted party guest' YouTube videos as metaphors – see Appendix 1). Used therapist self-disclosure of own self-critical thoughts in order to demonstrate the fallacy of 'healthy normality' (e.g., 'you're a terrible therapist!').

- Aaron practiced **mindfulness/metacognitive strategies** (e.g., STOP – 'stop', think', 'observe' and 'proceed') both within sessions and between sessions (with support worker input). He agreed to use self-monitoring and kept a thought diary, with twice-weekly electronic prompts from psychologist to compensate for his memory difficulties. For each thought, it was reinforced that we were less interested in reducing frequency but interested in increasing assessment of **'workability'** of thoughts and feelings (in service of personal values).

- Through these approaches, Aaron identified the following: 1. 'Over think things way too much'; 2. 'Paranoid about every step I take'; 3. 'Judge myself too much that's what holds me back, try not to care what people think about you'; 4. 'I keep trying to live the perfect life and body when nobody is perfect, everyone is different'; 5. 'Have a feeling that bad things could happen to me again and scared of them'; 6. 'Think into things a lot'; and 7. 'Think loads at night more than day; afraid of dying'.

- Aaron worked in sessions on defusing from unhelpful thoughts in sessions, and by planning future goals which are incompatible with these thoughts; including planning to purchase a car and drive again in the future. Used the **'naming the mind'** approach to reduce the power of these thoughts; This is a strategy in which naming the evaluative problem-solving mode of mind as if it were a separate entity supports defusion.[1]

- Focus on **'values identification'** aimed to support Aaron to focus not on what was difference since brain injury but what is ongoing (self-as-context). In addition to identifying these values, it was important to operationalise them in order to inform his actions. Aaron identified 1. 'Goodness' – 'Being good, kind, nice is the way to a peaceful unclouded soul. I'd rather help someone else than myself', 2. 'Love' – 'Love gives purpose and meaning to a person's actions/life. The emotion of love is one of the most fulfilling emotions. What are we without love?', and 3. 'Self-discipline' – 'To improve oneself, to do things correctly in life'. Regular review in sessions supported him to assess how consistent have actions been over the past day/week with identified values. In addition, rehabilitation goals were informed by his values which were then adopted by the MDT rehabilitation team, the most significant of which was to decide to continue his higher education and utilise his resources of time and energy on developing his social network and community activities.

- Developed alternative **'defusion'** strategies (cognitive and behavioural). Aaron acknowledged 'venting' as a previously used unhelpful coping strategy, however focused instead on values-consistent coping strategies, such as 'creativity', both in his artwork and in creative writing. He found motivational statements helpful in clarifying and reinforcing his values. For example, 'It's a rough road that leads to greatness'; 'I can entertain thoughts without accepting them'; 'snakes are not really there' (thoughts are fleeting intangible phenomena).

Outcome

Aaron reported that he found the ACT approach engaging and interesting; his strengths in verbal comprehension and language were helpful for success of more abstract interventions (translating values and preferences into concrete goals).

Significant executive difficulties were successfully accommodated through personally tailored external structures and memory aids (supporting the suggestion that difficulties with cognitive flexibility need not be a barrier to achieving greater psychological flexibility). Psychological process and outcome measures showed that, during the period of assessment, although standardised scores of anxiety and depression remained within the same clinical ranges (see Graph 2.1), with 'mild' depressive symptoms and 'moderate' anxiety symptoms using the Hospital Anxiety and Depression Scale (HADS: Zigmond & Snaith, 1983), there was a reduction in the assessment of psychological flexibility (see Graph 2.2) on the Acceptance and Action Questionnaire (Hayes et al., 2004); the 2nd edition (AAQ-II) was used, which is considered a general measure of psychological flexibility (see Bond et al., 2011).[2] Given that a central tenet of therapy was to undermine avoidance and distraction in the face of difficult emotions, it might be expected that anxiety would be experienced, as reliance on these ultimately unhelpful coping strategies is reduced. Aaron agreed to work with rehabilitation support systems and recommenced his university course, and no further incidents of venting of verbal aggression have been recorded to date. It is also the case that some anxiety may be engendered by the therapy itself in the short term. By definition, reducing reliance on ultimately unhelpful coping strategies such as distraction and avoidance is likely to produce psychological discomfort. In summary, the ACT approach was useful in support Aaron to address the neuropsychological barriers to achieving further progress with his MDT rehabilitation goals, in accordance with his personal values. This major goal of ACT of

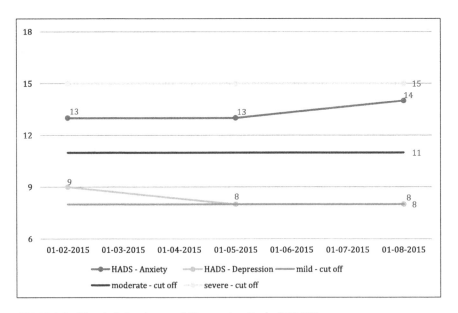

GRAPH 2.1 Hospital Anxiety and Depression Scale (HADS) scores

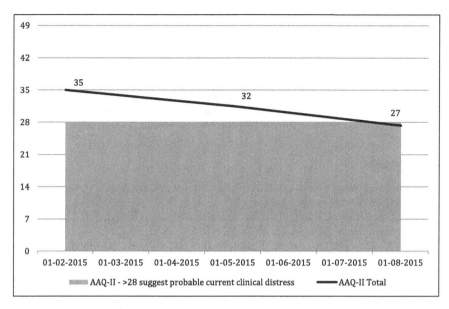

GRAPH 2.2 Acceptance and Action Questionnaire – 2nd edition (AAQ-II) scores

improving functioning and engagement in meaningful life providing a good fit with neurorehabilitation following brain injury.

Conclusion

The current case example is provided to for illustrative purposes of delivery of an ACT approach following brain injury and meets limited criteria for rating scales for quality rating scales of n-of-1 trials (RoBiNT: Tate et al., 2013). In addition, the change in scores on the AAQ-II has a Reliable Change Index (RCI) of −1.1, which is not statistically significant.[3] However, in ACT, as with brain injury rehabilitation, the desired outcome is often increased participation. It appears to the authors that psychological flexibility may be best conceptualised as a dynamic psychological process that is not easily captured by static, self-report measures. The contextual nature of MDT working as part of a neurorehabilitation team approach to achieving functional goals is are therefore relevant measures of success and support integrative and interdisciplinary work between all rehabilitation professionals working with people after brain injury. Aaron himself reported satisfaction with the ACT approach, the flexible nature of the structure of the work and the multimodal approach, as opposed to exclusively paper-and-pen exercises, was reported as a relief as he took a break from higher education. Aaron said that the main focus which he took away from our work was to 'be present in my life, take what my mind says with a pinch of salt, and not avoid the things I care about'.

Notes

1 Hayes et al. (2003) suggest that if 'naming the mind' does not seem to fit the client's personal style, it could be given a descriptive label such as the 'Reactive Mind'.
2 There is also the Acceptance and Action Questionnaire – Acquired Brain Injury (Sylvester, 2011). The decision to use the AAQ-ABI or the AAQ-II in an ABI population requires consideration of the targeted outcome (Whiting et al., 2015).
3 See Jacobson and Truax (1991) for calculation of Reliable Change Index (RCI), and Bond et al. (2011) for psychometric properties of the AAQ-II.

References

American Psychiatric Association. (2013). *Diagnostic and statistical manual of mental disorders* (5th ed.). Washington, DC: Author.

Anson, K., & Ponsford, J. L. (2006). Evaluation of a coping skills group following traumatic brain injury. *Brain Injury, 20*(2), 167–178.

Bond, F. W., Hayes, S. C., Baer, R. A., Carpenter, K. C., Guenole, N., Orcutt, H. K. . . . Zettle, R. D. (2011). Preliminary psychometric properties of the Acceptance and Action Questionnaire – II: A revised measure of psychological flexibility and acceptance. *Behavior Therapy, 42*, 676–688.

Ciarrochi, J., & Bailey, A. (2008). *A CBT-practitioner's guide to ACT: How to bridge the gap between cognitive behavioral therapy and acceptance and commitment therapy*. Oakland, CA: New Harbinger Publications.

Harris, R. (2007). *The happiness trap: Stop struggling, start living*. Wollombi, New South Wales: Exisle Publishing Limited.

Harris, R., & Hayes, S. C. (2009). *Act made simple*. New York: New Harbinger Publications.

Hayes, S. C., Luoma, J. B., Bond, F. W., Masuda, A., & Lillis, J. (2006). Acceptance and Commitment Therapy: Model, processes, and outcomes. *Behaviour Research and Therapy, 44*(1), 1–25.

Hayes, S. C., Strosahl, K. D., & Wilson, K. G. (2003). *Acceptance and commitment therapy: An experiential approach to behavior change*. New York: Guilford Press.

Hayes, S. C., Strosahl, K. D., Wilson, K. G., Bissett, R. T., Pistorello, J., Toarmino, D. . . . McCurry, S. M. (2004). Measuring experiential avoidance: A preliminary test of a working model. *Psychological Record, 54*(4), 553–578.

Jacobson, N. S., & Truax, P. (1991). Clinical significance: A statistical approach to defining meaningful change in psychotherapy research. *Journal of Consulting and Clinical Psychology, 59*(1), 12–19.

Kabat-Zinn, J. (1994). *Wherever you go, there you are: Mindfulness meditation in everyday life*. New York: Hyperion.

Kangas, M., & McDonald, S. (2011). Is it time to act? The potential of acceptance and commitment therapy for psychological problems following acquired brain injury. *Neuropsychological Rehabilitation, 21*(2), 250–276.

Kim, C., Johnson, N. F., Cilles, S. E., & Gold, B. T. (2011). Common and distinct mechanisms of cognitive flexibility in prefrontal cortex. *The Journal of Neuroscience, 31*(13), 4771–4779.

Myles, S. M. (2004). Understanding and treating loss of sense of self following brain injury: A behavior analytic approach. *International Journal of Psychology and Psychological Therapy, 4*(3), 487–504.

Pinker, S. (1997). *How the mind works*. New York: W. W. Norton & Company.

Simpson, G. K., Tate, R. L., Whiting, D. L., & Cotter, R. E. (2011). Suicide prevention after traumatic brain injury: A randomized controlled trial of a program for the psychological treatment of hopelessness. *The Journal of Head Trauma Rehabilitation, 26*(4), 290–300.

Soo, C., Tate, R. L., & Lane-Brown, A. (2011). A systematic review of Acceptance and Commitment Therapy (ACT) for managing anxiety: Applicability for people with acquired brain injury? *Brain Impairment, 12*(1), 54–70.

Sylvester, M. (2011). *Acceptance and commitment therapy for improving adaptive functioning in persons with a history of pediatric acquired brain injury.* (Doctor of Philosophy in Clinical Psychology Dissertation), University of Nevada, Reno.

Tate, R. L., Perdices, M., Rosenkoetter, U., Wakim, D., Godbee, K., Togher, L., & McDonald, S. (2013). Revision of a method quality rating scale for single-case experimental designs and n-of-1 trials: The 15-item risk of bias in N-of-1 trials (RoBiNT) scale. *Neuropsychological Rehabilitation, 23*(5), 619–638.

Törneke, N. (2010). *Learning RFT: An introduction to relational frame theory and its clinical application.* Oakland, CA: New Harbinger Publications.

Whiting, D. L., Deane, F. P., Ciarrochi, J., McLeod, H. J., & Simpson, G. K. (2015). Validating measures of psychological flexibility in a population with acquired brain injury. *Psychological Assessment, 27*(2), 415–423.

Whiting, D. L., Deane, F. P., Simpson, G. K., Ciarrochi, J., & McLeod, H. J. (2017). Acceptance and commitment therapy delivered in a dyad after a severe traumatic brain injury: A feasibility study. *Clinical Psychologist, 22*(2), 230–240.

Whiting, D. L., Deane, F. P., Simpson, G. K., McLeod, H. J., & Ciarrochi, J. (2017). Cognitive and psychological flexibility after a traumatic brain injury and the implications for treatment in acceptance-based therapies: A conceptual review. *Neuropsychological Rehabilitation, 27*(2), 263–299.

Whiting, D. L., Simpson, G. K., Ciarrochi, J., & McLeod, H. J. (2012). Assessing the feasibility of Acceptance and Commitment Therapy in promoting psychological adjustment after severe traumatic brain injury. *Brain Injury, 26*(4–5), 588–589.

Wilson, B. A., Evans, J. J., & Gracey, F. (2009). Goal setting as a way of planning and evaluating neuropsychological rehabilitation. In B. Wilson, F. Gracey, J. Evans, & A. Bateman (Eds.), *Neuropsychological rehabilitation: Theory, models, therapy and outcome* (pp. 37–46). Cambridge: Cambridge University Press.

Wilson, K. G., Sandoz, E. K., & Kitchens, J. (2010). The Valued Living Questionnaire: Defining and measuring valued action within a behavioral framework. *The Psychological Record, 60*, 249–272.

Ylvisaker, M., McPherson, K., Kayes, N., & Pellett, E. (2008). Metaphoric identity mapping: Facilitating goal setting and engagement in rehabilitation after traumatic brain injury. *Neuropsychological Rehabilitation, 18*, 713–741.

Zigmond, A. S., & Snaith, R. P. (1983). The hospital anxiety and depression scale. *Acta Psychiatrica Scandinavica, 67*, 361–370.

APPENDIX 1

Useful information on ACT resources

Examples of metaphors and exercises corresponding with the core therapeutic processes of ACT

Acceptance and willingness

Explore the costs of control, whilst introducing acceptance and willingness as alternatives, e.g.:

- 'Don't think about chocolate cake' – paradoxical increase in the thought by conscious struggle.
- 'Old Joe at the party' – the problems with strict rule following and attempted control of those things beyond our sphere of influence.
- 'Being Willingly Out of Breath' – willing acceptance of unpleasant sensations.
- 'Quicksand' – the struggle for control causes further problems and distress.

Cognitive defusion

Disentangle from our self-talk and observe cognitions as just words, entities separate from ourselves, e.g.:

- 'Floating leaves on a moving stream' – stepping back and observing thoughts.
- 'Your mind is not your friend' – creating a degree of separation from our unhelpful thoughts from ourselves (also 'naming the mind' or 'reactive mind').
- 'Milk, milk, milk. . . .' – exercise aimed at deliteralising language.
- 'The Master Storyteller' – explains the constant narrative, of our minds, including judgements, predictions, and evaluations (also the 'don't get eaten' machine).

Contact with the present moment

As practiced through mindfulness exercises ('paying attention in a particular way: on purpose, in the present moment, and nonjudgementally' Kabat-Zinn, 1994), e.g.:

- Engage clients in adapting the exercises to fit their own needs and situations. Following brain injury, it can be helpful to shorten guided exercises, and involve regular daily activities.
- Practice present-moment awareness in sessions, especially when discussing painful emotions or memories ('what's happening for you right now?').
- Responding to triggers – useful practice to support managing impulsive behaviours following acquired neurological conditions.

Self-as-context

Support the client to take a different perspective on the self, e.g.:

- 'The Chessboard' – facilitate a shift in perspective from self-as-content to self-as-context.
- 'The Prince and the Beggar' – the continuity of an identity that remains stable even through changing circumstances.
- 'Taking off your Armor' – useful for clients with a history of trauma who have become attached to a conceptualised self that is guarded and untrusting yet who value closeness and intimacy.

Values

Values are personally important and meaningful and enable a life of purpose and engagement. They are not goals; they support the identification of goals, e.g.:

- 'The classroom professor and the large empty jar' – the prioritisation of values and balancing what is really important to us.
- 'What do you want your life to stand for?' – for instance the autobiography or tombstone.
- Use of ACT process measures, such as the Valued Living Questionnaire (Wilson, Sandoz, & Kitchens, 2010); The Survey of Life Principles Version 2.2 – Card Sorting Task (CST; Ciarrochi & Bailey, 2008).

Committed action

Active and purposeful engagement in behaviour that is consistent with a person's values, consistent with goal-setting in the process of neurorehabilitation, e.g.:

- 'Passengers on the bus' – focusing on moving in a valued direction and not stopping to be distracted by unhelpful thoughts, feelings and experiences.

- 'The rope bridge' – it is not possible to find out if the bridge is safe or not whilst standing still, and fear must not impede our progress.
- 'The bicycle factory' – the manager needs to get involved, despite the team-work required, ensuring dependence on others is not fostered. Useful for relapse prevention and building larger patterns of committed action in the long-term management of an acquired neurological condition.

Freely available ACT resources

The ACT community is known for freely sharing resources, including videos, manuals, e-books and papers that are available. Here are some examples of websites with useful and freely available resources:

- The Association for Contextual Behavioral Science (ACBS; https://contextual science.org)
- Contextual Consulting (https://contextualconsulting.co.uk)
- Russ Harris's work (www.actmindfully.com.au, https://thehappinesstrap. com/free-resources/, https://imlearningact.com/free-resources/)
- Portland Psychotherapy Clinic (http://portlandpsychotherapyclinic.com)
- Positive Psychology Programme (https://positivepsychologyprogram.com/ act-acceptance-and-commitment-therapy)
- Books published by New Harbinger provide free companion resources

APPENDIX 2

Suggested therapy modifications in ACT to account for cognitive impairments (adapted from Whiting, Deane, Simpson, McLeod et al., 2017)

- Shorten length of the sessions
- Using memory aids, e.g., written notes, cue cards, recordings
- Simplification of tasks
- Increased frequency of sessions
- Summarising and reviewing content regularly
- Focus on behavioural techniques
- Involve a family member in the therapy process
- Initial sessions focus on educating, normalising and validating
- Training to enhance other skills, e.g., social skills
- Concrete examples as opposed to abstract
- Modelling of assignments by therapist and client
- Repetition and slowed presentation
- Being directive in the discussions and with therapy
- Using personally relevant and concrete metaphors
- Engaging in experiential exercises including role playing
- Defusion techniques that are concrete, e.g., physicalising the thought
- Focus on behavioural activation components
- Providing tangible ideas, e.g., Card Sorting Task from the Survey of Life Principles 2.2 (Ciarrochi & Bailey, 2008)
- Promotion of values-based, goal-directed behaviour
- Shorter mindfulness exercises
- Allowing client to develop their own meaning from metaphors

3

MINDFULNESS IN NEUROLOGICAL CONDITIONS

Niels Detert

How do you cope with the experience of disability, of losses in multiple domains of life, of frustrating limitations in the long term, of difficult symptoms and pain and in some cases of a deteriorating prognosis? How do you manage the intense emotions which naturally arise with this experience? How do you regulate the anxiety which arises in reaction to these emotions? How do you respond when old coping strategies are overwhelmed, outdated or disabled? How do you manage anxiogenic and depressogenic mental processes such as worry, rumination and negative thoughts? How can you change your way of life to balance the demands of self-care with the demands of family, work and society? How can you find meaning, appreciation and joy in life? These are some of the urgent problems which face people with a neuro-disability or neurological disease and with which mindfulness training offers a way of working. Rather than merely a treatment for depression and anxiety (although it is that), or specific advice for specific problems, the intention is to give people a tool, a way of meeting their own unique and unpredictable life experience moment by moment and responding wisely, kindly and skilfully to reduce stress, anxiety and depression and where possible to find meaning, appreciation and joy. In my experience, and in the emerging evidence, this is borne out, and although mindfulness training is no magic cure and is probably as effective as other therapies in reducing symptoms of depression and anxiety in the short term, it does promise a way of working with these challenges which is suitable for a range of people in a resource-efficient way, and provides people with a long-term coping strategy, and indeed a method for ongoing development, which goes beyond symptom reduction and offers people a foundation for building new ways of coping with their changed and changing situation.

Theory and practice

Mindfulness has been described as 'the awareness that emerges through paying attention on purpose, in the present moment, and non-judgementally to things as they are' (Williams, Teasdale, Segal, & Kabat-Zinn, 2007, p. 47). It is considered to be a capacity that is already present in people, and which people possess dispositionally to varying degrees, but which is underdeveloped and can be trained. The training is by daily formal periods of practicing paying attention in this way and then applying this developing capacity for awareness in everyday life situations. Several clinical interventional programmes have been developed to train mindfulness, including eight-week group courses such as Mindfulness Based Stress Reduction (MBSR), Mindfulness Based Cognitive Therapy (MBCT) and the 'Breathworks' programme developed in the UK, as well as adaptations for particular populations (e.g., Mindfulness Based Relapse Prevention in addictions, MBRP, Bowen, Chawla, & Marlatt, 2010). These programmes have also been adapted into web-based, book and audio formats for independent training. In addition, elements of mindfulness practice have been incorporated into other formal individual therapies as components of a broader package, such as in Acceptance and Commitment Therapy (ACT) and in Dialectical Behaviour Therapy (DBT) and informally in other therapies. In this chapter I will focus on the use of MBSR and MBCT.

Eight-week mindfulness programmes are run with group sizes of ten to 20, sometimes more or less, with weekly sessions of 90–180 minutes and 45–60 minutes of home practice using audio-recorded guidance. During sessions there is live guidance of mindfulness practices, followed by instructor-led exploration of participants' experiences during the practice, modelling qualitative characteristics of mindfulness (nonreactive, nonjudgemental observation and exploration of experience), drawing out learning points and giving practical advice. There are further discussions, with an experiential focus, of home practice and a curriculum of psycho-educational topics including further experiential exercises and mindfulness practices.

Historically MBSR was the original programme, developed by Jon Kabat-Zinn in the 1980s, based on techniques from Buddhist meditation and yoga and applied initially in helping patients with physical health conditions and especially chronic pain. MBCT was developed by Zindel Segal, Mark Williams and John Teasdale during the 1990s (2002, 2013), originally as a theory-driven intervention for preventing relapse in recurrent depression. Both have been applied more widely to a diversity of conditions and populations with a maturing evidence base summarised here. MBSR and MBCT share the same core mindfulness practices, with the addition of a couple of further adaptations in MBCT. The curriculum in both focuses on development of core mindfulness skills in the first three weeks using practices focusing on awareness of body sensations, and sensations of breathing and movement. In weeks 4 and 5 there is a focus on using these developing skills to observe the reaction of aversion to unpleasant experiences and using mindful awareness to decouple the link between unpleasant experience and reactive habits of thought and action which may worsen anxiety, stress and low mood, and to open up the possibility of responding in more appropriate, effective and kindly ways. The further curriculum varies somewhat depending on the particular format. MBSR focuses on applying mindful awareness as a way of working with stress reactions in a variety of aspects of life, such as physical pain, emotional distress, personal relationships and time stress for example. MBCT focuses on observing the process of thoughts, feelings and activity, the links between these and stress/anxiety/mood and applying alternative mindful responses to cope with difficult experiences. In theory these techniques target common causal pathways of anxiety, stress and depression, and therefore they provide a general-purpose way of working with psychological distress triggered in reaction to diverse problematic experiences and life circumstances.

In practice the procedure of mindfulness training is very simple. Each type of meditation practiced has an experiential focus (such as breath, body sensations, sounds, thoughts, feelings, open awareness), and the instruction is to place attention on that focus and maintain it. When one notices the attention has wandered, the instruction is simply to bring it back to the focus without judgement and continue. This deceptively simple procedure has some far-reaching aims. It trains attention to be more stable and flexible. It throws into relief the distracting thoughts which arise in the mind and opens the possibility of beginning to notice the thought process. This opens the possibility of observing the negative effects of thoughts on mood, especially judgemental thoughts, and the ways in which our experience is overlaid with a layer of concepts, so that a simple experience becomes coloured or distorted in sometimes unhelpful ways (e.g., an intense sensation becomes 'unbearable'). Practicing observing the thought process enables the possibility of 'decentering', i.e., not identifying with thoughts, not seeing them as real, true in themselves or imperative, but just thoughts, events in the mind which come and go, and which we can choose whether or not to respond to or believe. There is the opportunity to practice relating to experience as it is, unframed by thoughts, and to find a new way to manage difficult experiences, bringing kindness and care rather than aversion and self-judgement. There is also the possibility to observe and become aware of long-standing problematic patterns and make new choices as situations arise.

For a practical example of these principles in action I recommend reading the transcript from the case example at the end of the chapter.

Evidence

There is an increasingly mature body of published literature from which to draw conclusions about the effectiveness of mindfulness-based interventions (MBIs) and recent systematic reviews and meta-analyses have synthesised the evidence in different populations. Piet and Hougaard (2011), in a systematic review and meta-analysis of six large randomised controlled trials (RCTs), found that MBCT is more effective than treatment as usual or placebo control in preventing depressive relapse in nondepressed people with three or more previous episodes and in two studies was at least as good as maintenance anti-depressants. In a review of reviews, Gotink et al. (2015) performed a systematic review and meta-analysis of 23 reviews of randomised controlled trials (RCTs), encompassing 115 unique RCTs and 8683 patients, in diverse clinical populations, including depression, anxiety, cancer, cardiovascular disease and chronic pain; they found small to medium effects on clinical outcomes (Depression, Cohen's $d = 0.37$; Anxiety, $d = 0.49$; Stress, $d = 0.51$; Quality of life, $d = 0.39$; physical functioning, $d = 0.27$).[1] Strauss, Cavanagh, Oliver, and Pettman (2014) examined a more selected sub-group of RCTs with participants with a current primary diagnosis of depression or a formal anxiety disorder. They found, with inactive controls, a medium effect on depression symptom severity, but not anxiety, although the confidence interval overlap with zero effect is small. However, in a systematic review and meta-analysis of effects of meditation on anxiety (Chen et al., 2012), though drawn more broadly than the Strauss review to include anxiety symptoms and not specifically anxiety disorders, there were medium effects in 11 RCTs of MBSR and MBCT.

In neurological populations, there is evidence in multiple sclerosis (MS), epilepsy, Parkinson's disease (PD), traumatic brain injury (TBI), stroke and pilot work in aphasia and nonepileptic attacks.

The MS literature includes two RCTs of MBSR in comparison with treatment as usual (Grossman et al., 2010; Kolahkaj & Zargar, 2015), a wait-list RCT (Simpson, 2017; Simpson et al., 2018), a waiting list controlled trial of MBCT (Hoogerwerf, Bol, Lobbestael, Hupperts, & Van Heugten, 2017) and two smaller controlled trials of nonstandardised programmes focusing more on mindful movement and introducing elements of Tai Chi/Chi Gong (Tavee, Rense, Planchon, Butler, & Stone, 2011; Mills & Allen, 2000). A further controlled trial used Tai Chi alone in weekly 90 minute sessions for six months (Burschka, Keune, Oy, Oschmann, & Kuhn, 2014). All of these found beneficial effects in line with the literature in anxiety and depression, quality of life and on some physical measures, including particularly fatigue. An RCT of an online MS-specific mindfulness course was effective in the short-term but group differences disappeared at the six-month follow up (Cavalera et al., 2019).

Of interest, trait mindfulness in MS has been associated with a number of benefits in correlational studies, in perceived stress and resilience (Senders, Bourdette, Hanes, Yadav, & Shinto, 2014), in reduced pain experience (Senders, Borgatti, Hanes, & Shonto, 2018) and in attachment style (Mohamadirizi, Shaygannejad, & Mohamadirizi, 2017). In another paradigm, following a randomised controlled trial of an online mindfulness course, a correlation was found between mindfulness and quality of life, anxiety, depression, fatigue and sleep over follow up assessments (Pagnini et al., 2019). Bogosian, Hughes, Norton, Silber, and

Moss-Morris (2016) found that decentring and self-efficacy had large mediating effects, with acceptance and self-compassion developing more gradually over a longer period. Crescentinin and colleagues (2018) in a small controlled study in MS, found changes in personality traits following mindfulness training, with an increase in character traits reflecting maturity of the self at the interpersonal (self-directedness) and interpersonal (cooperativeness) levels, and decreased trait anxiety.

In epilepsy two RCTs have demonstrated effectiveness (Tang, Poon, & Kwan, 2015; Thompson et al., 2015), and of particular interest, Tang and colleagues' study provided evidence of reduced seizure frequency. Also of interest, an RCT comparing progressive muscle relaxation (PMR) and a focused attention control (Haut et al., 2018), found both treatments effective in reducing seizure frequency in treatment resistant epilepsy, with greater stress reduction in the PMR group, and, whilst the focused attention condition was very much more limited than mindfulness training, these findings support the hypothesis that stress reducing and relaxing treatments are effective, and it would be interesting to compare MBCT or MBSR with PMR.

In Parkinson's disease (PD), there is preliminary data from several small studies (Pickut et al., 2013, 2015; Dissanayaka et al., 2016; Fitzpatrick, Simpson, & Smith, 2010), broadly showing benefits but with heterogeneity of outcomes, and one of these showed no benefit on depression (Pickut et al., 2015). A wait-list controlled RCT in PD used a nonstandard six-session intervention with emphasis on lifestyle advice combined with mindfulness practice and showed small effects on measures of stress, mindfulness and activities of daily living (Advocat et al., 2016).

In traumatic brain injury (TBI) Bedard et al., having previously reported positive pilot data (2012), carried out a randomised controlled trial in comparison with a waiting list control with 38 patients in each arm (2013), and they found a medium effect size on depressive symptom severity.

In nonepileptic attacks there is some very preliminary but interesting work reported by Baslet, Dworetzky, Perez, and Oser (2015) in the form of a case series of six patients given one-to-one mindfulness training. The current author's own experience with patients with nonepileptic seizures completing MBCT is of reduced seizure frequency in a substantial proportion, with complete remission a less common outcome. The wider literature on the use of mindfulness in somatoform disorders provides evidence of some benefit (e.g., van Ravesteijn, Lucassen, Bor, van Weel, & Speckens, 2013, in mixed somatoform disorders; Schmidt et al., 2011; Grossman, Tiefenthaler-Gilmer, Raysz, & Kesper, 2007, in fibromyalgia), but further research is needed. In an uncontrolled study of a clinical sample of mixed neurological diagnoses (n = 98) Detert and Douglass (2014) showed medium pre-post effects on depression/anxiety and large effects on perceived stress, supporting the stress-coping rationale of mindfulness training.

In aphasia some pilot work with small numbers and single cases have been reported, and demonstrate feasibility at least, but these have used a nonstandard five-day (Marshall, Laures-Gore, & Love, 2018; Laures-Gore & Marshall, 2016, case study), or four-week training (Dickinson, Friary, & McCann, 2017, case study).

There is evidence of cognitive benefit from mindfulness training in non-brain-injured populations (e.g., Jensen, Vangkilde, Frokjaer, & Hasselbalch, 2012; Chiesa, Calati, & Serretti, 2011; van Vugt, 2015; Schöne, Gruber, Graetz Bernhof, & Malinowski, 2018). In neuro populations there is some limited and some inconclusive evidence of cognitive benefit with a null result from a high-quality study of a limited attention training intervention, substantially briefer and not comparable in quality to mindfulness training (McMillan, Robertson, Brock, & Chorlton, 2002), and some positive results from three smaller studies; first, a controlled trial of MBSR in TBI and Stroke (Johansson, Bjuhr, & Rönnbäck, 2012), which also demonstrated reduced fatigue in the long-term, second, a randomised controlled trial of phone telehealth mindfulness training, versus initial mindfulness instructions only, in MS (Frontario, Sherman, Krupp, & Charvet, 2016), which also demonstrated improvements to mood, and third, an experimental study (McHugh & Wood, 2013). Confidence in the evidence of the effect on fatigue is supported by a meta-analysis showing a small effect size over four studies in TBI, stroke and MS (Ulrichsen et al., 2016). There are some inconclusive results from uncontrolled pilot studies on cognition in neurological disease with significant design limitations (Blankespoor, Schellekens, Vos, Speckens, & de Jong, 2017; Cash, Ekouevi, Kilbourn, & Lageman, 2016). A key unanswered question is whether the cognitive and fatigue benefits are independent of improvements to mood.

Adapting mindfulness training in a neuro population

Adaptation of mindfulness-based interventions in a neuro population depends very much on the needs of individuals. The simple and repetitive nature of mindfulness practice places less cognitive demand on patients in comparison with other therapies and provides a substantial degree of structure in the form of guided practices. During mindful movement practices because the focus is on mindfulness rather than specific movements, physical aspects of practice can be adjusted to suit people's physical ability. In general people with mild to moderate cognitive and/or physical impairment will require relatively little adaptation, and these adaptations can be managed in a group.

Some general adaptations include reviewing and editing written course materials and adjusting the physical practices. MBCT and its course materials were originally designed for people with recurrent depression, but the course materials are relatively easily adaptable to a physical health or neuro population with some small edits. The body scan practice can be done lying down, sitting or in other postures as appropriate to individuals. When doing mindful movement in a group with balance problems or fatigue, long standing practices can be avoided, and the emphasis can be on floor- or chair-based practices. For people in wheelchairs, upper body practices can be done from sitting and these can be done with a mixed ability group with some people sitting and some standing. More extensive sequences of hatha yoga postures can be adjusted to include some which can be attempted by all, and some in which some group members will omit movements and practice mindfulness of breathing, or of course could be omitted altogether. Where someone has specific difficulties which could be managed better with a carer present then carers can be included in the group and ideally should commit to their own mindfulness practice.

A severe degree of cognitive impairment may require individual adaptation and suitability should be carefully considered. Use of small group numbers or individual sessions, and inclusion of carers can be considered. People with more severe executive dysfunction face the same problems as with other interventions in initiating and monitoring their own practice and applying mindfulness in everyday life. If someone finds it difficult to self-initiate and self-monitor home mindfulness practice then this could be supported in the usual ways, with strategies such as alarms and reminders, or with the help of a carer, who ideally would also participate on the course. People with more severe memory problems may find mindfulness training relatively possible in comparison with other therapies as the memory load is light in the experiential elements of the course, although it will be harder for them to benefit from more conceptual elements of the curriculum. Nevertheless, remembering home practice and what they are doing may be a challenge and if needed they may also benefit from the support of a carer who does the course and the practice at the same time. Severe aphasia would likely prevent effective participation on a standard mindfulness course, although other modalities of mindful movement such as yoga or practices of Qi Gong/Tai Qi could be considered as partial alternatives. Even so, there are case reports of people with some degree of dysphasia having successfully made use of mindfulness training (Orenstein, Basilakos, & Marshall, 2012).

With whom does it work best? Indications, contra-indications and challenges

There can be a variety of possible indications for MBCT/MBSR. The most obvious are to use it as a treatment for current depression, anxiety and stress, as a preventative treatment for recurrent depression, and as a long-term method for stress coping. Even in the absence of current depression or anxiety there is a rationale to use it as a method of coping with long-term neurological conditions that are likely to deteriorate or relapse, or that are stable but present ongoing challenges. It has a use in developing skills of emotion awareness and regulation, either in people who have a psycho-developmental weakness in this area due to problematic childhood experiences or in people who have acquired emotion dysregulation through a brain injury or illness. It can have a further use in supporting change of problematic patterns of response and coping by enabling observation of habitual patterns and providing a method for pausing habitual reactivity and selecting more functional responses.

There is a dose-response relationship between mindfulness practice and outcome (Gotink et al., 2015). Accordingly, factors that affect home practice are significant determinants of outcome. Strong motivation is a positive factor and would be a reason to consider mindfulness training even in the presence of other problematic factors. Ambivalent motivation would a be a reason to consider not recommending mindfulness training or to have an open discussion about motivation.

Practical considerations are very important. Travel logistics may prevent some people from attending and should be considered. People who have busy lives with little spare time or a lot of family and work duties will naturally find it harder, and some discussion about this is necessary. In such cases motivation to make the time is key. Shorter home practices can be considered.

The people who have the most difficulty are those who use busyness as a coping strategy, either as a way of controlling their lives or as a way of avoiding feelings. People with such a coping style have usually maintained their busy pattern when faced with the challenges of a brain injury/condition and the disability, fatigue and stress that comes with it, creating a vicious circle of stress and fatigue and leaving no space for anything else, including mindfulness practice. There is a risk that such people attend the course but never do their home practice, either dropping out halfway through or reaching the end without much benefit except for the group experience, possibly disappointed or even discouraged about psychological approaches, self-critical or even feeling worse. This should be anticipated in the assessment interview, formulating the pattern of busyness, addressing the question of motivation and willingness to set aside the habitual pattern of busyness for the course and problem-solving how to fit in the home practice.

People with previous experience of psychological trauma can benefit from mindfulness training (see Banks, Newman, & Saleem, 2015 for a review), but some adjustments of emphasis need to be made in delivery of the course to maintain safety from excessive trauma re-experiencing. The usual mindfulness instructions convey an initial message of allowing experience to be as it is and accepting all experiences (inner and outer) equally, in order to cut through habitual reactions of aversion. These instructions are refined during the course to include the idea of appropriate responding to experience. Initial instructions can be understood to imply the indiscriminate invitation of all experiences into consciousness, and this needs specific clarification for people with trauma experiences. With the arising of trauma memories or overwhelming thoughts/feelings which are harmful, some more active protective response is needed, and skilful responses include using mindful sensory grounding to direct attention into something neutral in the present moment. Likewise, a specific adjustment is needed for the 'Working with Difficulty' practice in week five of the course, in which a difficulty is deliberately recalled, just to make clear that participants should select some issue of medium difficulty, not something traumatic or overwhelming.

In formal anxiety disorders, careful consideration should be given to whether mindfulness training is an appropriate treatment, given the weak evidence on this at present. If the formulation suggests that there are established habitual patterns of avoidance and specific structures of belief that will need challenging and restructuring, and there is not clear insight and strong motivation but weak insight, ambivalence or resistance. Then a one-to-one therapy will be better indicated, though mindfulness training might be considered as an adjunct before or after therapy if appropriate.

There is a high proportion of people with functional disorders in neurological populations, and evidence is limited. In my experience, with appropriate cautions there is no reason in principle to exclude such patients from mindfulness courses, but it is important to manage expectations of symptomatic outcomes (except in nonepileptic attacks). It is unlikely in my experience that there will be symptomatic benefit in functional motor and sensory symptoms from a mindfulness course alone, although there may be benefit in some cases, and this is more likely if the symptom is paroxysmal, clearly stress sensitive or is itself a manifestation of anxiety. In our pre-post study (Detert & Douglass, 2014) the small subgroup of patients with functional neurological conditions (16 out of 98) showed only a small effect on measures of anxiety and depression, significantly less than other neurological groups, but it did show a very large effect in perceived stress coping, which was not statistically different from other neurological patients. Accordingly the rationale in many functional cases would be to cope better with the stress of chronic symptoms or as a helpful adjunct to therapy. There is also a theoretical risk of mindfulness acting to maintain or exacerbate functional motor and sensory symptoms, given the emerging consensus on the role of abnormal symptom-focused attention in functional symptoms (Edwards, Adams, Brown, Pareés, & Friston, 2012), and whilst further research is needed on the interaction of mindfulness training with functional disorders, it is reasonable to give instructions not to focus excessively on functional symptoms in the practice but instead to use mindfulness of other aspects of experience. Finally, there is a theoretical rationale that doing this may contribute to better managing and maybe reducing functional symptoms, and indeed effective physiotherapy treatments of functional movement disorders include specific attentional interventions, i.e., distracting the patient's attention from their movements whilst retraining normal movements (Nielsen et al., 2015).

My reflections on using mindfulness with people with neurological disorders

As I begin a new mindfulness course, I often remember something Jon Kabat-Zinn wrote about starting a new course, as I feel quite awed or daunted by what we are trying to do by the amount of suffering in the room and by the apparently flimsy answer I have of practicing awareness and letting experience be. It is usual for people to be sceptical, or at least not to understand how this activity is going to help them, and of course they are soon, rightly, disillusioned of any hopes of clearing the mind or of blissful meditative states, although in fact many people do experience the meditation as relaxing. As the course goes on it emerges that what is on offer is both much more ordinary than expected, in that it involves grappling with and immersing oneself in the stresses and experiences of everyday life, and much more revolutionary than expected, in that the training invites a shift of perspective on the whole of life experience. By about weeks four, five or six of the course I can see and hear that people are starting to 'get it' and beginning to feel a growing confidence in what they are doing. By the end of the course it is common to see people not only feeling better but hear them describing a sense of greater confidence in facing the future, linking this directly to the fact that they feel they have learned a way of dealing with stressful life events, which they can continue to apply and therefore feel emboldened and confident in facing adverse events in general. In a minority of cases people have described feeling better than they ever have, even before their illness, and most people who complete the course and practices describe at least some benefit, often significant. Participating in this journey is deeply rewarding, and of course there are other rewards, including the personal benefits of mindfulness practice for the teacher and the fact that it is an enjoyable activity for both participants and teacher, often enlivening rather than draining or tiring.

Practically speaking what I find particularly attractive about mindfulness training is that it is applicable to diverse difficulties and life situations, and this makes it feasible to offer as a general course to a wide range of patients, helping a greater number of people than could be achieved by one therapist doing one-to-one therapy in that time and achieving comparable results. The fact that it is resource efficient and that it is a method of coping rather than a treatment for a specific psychological disorder also makes it possible to include people who would not meet criteria for one-to-one therapy because they are not sufficiently depressed/anxious but who nevertheless experience a lot of life stress in facing disability and in some cases a deteriorating prognosis.

A case example

Referral and assessment

This lady in her early 60s with secondary progressive multiple sclerosis (MS), MS-related pain, fatigue and disability and marital difficulties was also suffering with symptoms of anxiety and possibly low mood, which were thought by her referring neurologist to be exacerbating the severity of her MS symptoms. Of particular interest, she reported that her pain was made worse by stress, by which it seemed that she meant both anxiety and angry feelings. On a questionnaire measure (Hospital Anxiety and Depression Scale, Zigmond, & Snaith, 1983) she scored at a high level for symptoms of anxiety and not depression, although I thought her mood was at least sub-optimal (Anxiety, 14/21; Depression, 0/21; clinical cut-offs at 11).

Formulation

My impression was that there were two main factors contributing to her experience of anxiety and angry feelings: her MS-related pain, fatigue and disability, and her conflictual interactions with her husband. In response to frustrating symptoms/disability and her husband, she was experiencing angry feelings and reacting to these angry feelings she was experiencing, which raised anxiety and left her engaging in cognitive self-attack/criticism, further increasing and not soothing her anxiety. This raised level of anxious arousal was in turn exacerbating her experience of pain in a vicious circle, and her ensuing distressed mental state and behaviour was possibly contributing to the systemic difficulty between her and her husband, or at least making it harder to manage. In terms of MBCT, the angry/fearful/anxious reaction is labelled aversion, and holds a key place in the MBCT model: some life experiences are unpleasant (or more accurately are appraised as unpleasant), and people experience an aversion reaction at those moments, which is then elaborated, exacerbated and maintained by cognitive interpretations and rumination, and by further cycles of aversion to the resulting unpleasant mental and physical states.

Mindfulness training seemed a good match for this pattern of difficulties, but I also considered the possibility that a one-to-one or couples approach might be needed in relation to the specific problems in her relationship. She opted for MBCT, and we decided to review the possibility of an onwards referral after that if needed.

Intervention and outcome

She completed the MBCT course and reported finding it very useful, continuing to practice post-course. Here I present a transcript from session 7 of the MBCT course in which key points of her formulation are drawn out and addressed. This episode is from a part of the session known as an inquiry, immediately after a mindfulness practice. In inquiries participants are invited to speak about their experience in the preceding practice, and the mindfulness teacher may answer questions or even give practical advice but particularly seeks to inquire further into peoples' experience, for example to explore and highlight processes of reactivity and aversion, and to model an experiential focus or an observing stance, decentring from thoughts and an interested nonjudgmental nonreactive nonstriving and kindly attitude. Of course there are about 20 people on the same course, and each person may only occasionally directly interact with the mindfulness teacher and is not necessarily expected to have an interaction of the depth of this example. It is expected that such interactions when they do occur will also be beneficial to others present, illustrating more widely applicable principles and insights.

During this conversation I, several times, checked her willingness to inquire further, as this inquiry does occur in the presence of the whole group. Her permission has also been sought and given to publish these details.

The focus in this passage is on exploring, clarifying and questioning the reactivity, which exacerbates and maintains anxiety and, for many people, depressed mood. Initially there is a focus on identifying the aversion (in the form of anger) to pain and exhaustion, and even the aversion/avoidance of the experience of anger in the form of self-attack. In the second part this is formulated, and an alternative mindful response is endorsed. Also of note, at the beginning of the passage she is reporting the discovery of an interesting and useful phenomenon – that she can affect her experience of her pain by where she chooses to put her attention and that when she puts her attention somewhere other than her body she does not feel her pain so much – a key tool in managing chronic pain.

PARTICIPANT: What I've noticed, for me, is that when, half way through, my pain goes completely, because I can't feel my body at all, but as soon as you wake me up as it were, bring me back to reality, it starts coming back again, it starts tingling and it starts tightening up.

THERAPIST: and what does that feel like?

P: I don't know what that means, I know that when I sleep I don't have pain, but I know that when I'm conscious of pain it makes it worse. So whether I'm looking for the pain whether it's there or not and I'm bringing it back I don't know.

T: During the practice, where's your attention?

P: Where's my attention, everywhere. First of all it's on my breathing and then it's in everything that hurts in my body, and then as I gradually um listen to more around me, I'm taken around me rather than in me. And I'm, I'm now, um, I think now I'm, I'm back in me, because I'm noticing all sorts of things that are happening in my body.

T: When you notice those things, what is going on in your feelings and thoughts?

P: Well for my thoughts, I can't remember my thoughts but what I feel at the moment is, is a little bit on the brink of tears. I think that's what I identify them as.

T: And what feeling is that?

P: I think if I looked at it logically I would say it's a feeling of exhaustion, because I know I'm exhausted.

T: So, there's exhaustion and there's pain.

P: Yes, and they always come together.

T: And then what's the feeling, about being exhausted and in pain?

P: Disappointment. Maybe anger, anger at myself.

T: Well, at any rate there's anger, but does it have to be at yourself?

P: Yes, because my anger's that I've allowed myself to get to this point of exhaustion.

[a section omitted here]

T: So there's an experience which is unpleasant, making it completely general it could be all kinds of different things, but in this case it's about exhaustion and pain. Then there's a reaction about not wanting it, that has anger in it.

P: Yeah.

T: Then actually there's not wanting the anger either.

P: Yes.

T: And so, various things happen to try and get away from the anger, and try and solve this problem including . . .

P: Blaming someone else.

T: Blaming someone else or instead of blaming someone else, blaming myself. Maybe if I blame myself that'll solve the problem. Maybe that'll get rid of the anger and the pain, but does it?

P: No, it just makes it worse. So what do you do, do you just . . .

T: So you notice those things that make it worse like self-critical thinking, the thoughts, you notice it's just thoughts.

P: They're not real.

Following the course she did not attend for a follow-up session, and I did not get information on the progress of her relationship difficulties, nor post-course questionnaire measures. However, in her end of course feedback and impact statement she wrote the following about the effects of the course on her life, demonstrating some good outcomes and the ongoing salience in her practice of the discoveries from the inquiry reported here and the course:

> I have learnt about myself, it has helped me to be in touch with my anger. It has taught me how to take time for myself and that I am worth it and how to do it. The course has given me knowledge on how to let thoughts come and then go without having to dwell on them. 'Thoughts are not facts' has been really an important realisation for me, especially those negative ones about myself. I can change them now more easily by relaxing, breathing and being kind to myself in words and thoughts. The course has helped me enjoy the here and now rather than rushing through life noticing nothing. I am a better person in my opinion because of the course.

In recent correspondence, kindly giving permission for her case to be used in this chapter, she wrote this about her ongoing mindfulness practice several years later:

> I continue to use mindfulness to calm myself even if it is only 3 mins in the chair. I find that stress, which I am not very good at, causes more pain and mindfulness relaxes me and helps to relax and decreases the pain. This has changed my life and has enabled me to be more positive about my condition and life in general.

Conclusion

Mindfulness-based interventions are effective evidence-based interventions for treating depression, managing anxiety, coping with the stress of illness and disability in the long term and exchanging outdated habitual patterns of behavioural/cognitive reaction for flexible situation-appropriate responding. In these respects, MBIs share many features with other therapies, although the course format enables a very resource-efficient therapy, and the theoretical rationale of addressing basic psychopathological mechanisms allows people with diverse problems to benefit in a single group. Mindfulness practice is of course not just a therapy for pathological mental states but provides a framework for personal development, change and life appreciation, which may be particularly relevant to people with neurological conditions needing to adapt to radically changed physical and cognitive circumstances or life expectations. These approaches have been shown to be feasible and appropriate in neurological populations with comparable results to other populations. Anecdotally, in this author's experience, these courses are also experienced as very enjoyable.

Note

1 A note on effect size: Cohen's *d* expresses the difference between two sample means in units of standard deviation. Hedges's *g* is a variation of Cohen's *d*, which corrects for biases due to small sample sizes. The magnitude of effect size can be interpreted in terms of the convention recommended by Cohen (1988): <0.2 is trivial, 0.2–0.5 is small, 0.5–0.8 is medium, ≥0.8 is large.

References

Advocat, J., Enticott, J., Vandenburg, B., Hassed, C., Hester, J., & Russell, G. (2016). The effects of a mindfulness-based lifestyle program for adults with Parkinson's disease: A mixed methods, wait list controlled randomised control study. *BMC Neurology, 16,* 166. https://doi.org/10.1186/s12883-016-0685-1

Banks, K., Newman, E., & Saleem, J. (2015). An overview of the research on mindfulness-based interventions for treating symptoms of posttraumatic stress disorder: A systematic review. *Journal of Clinical Psychology, 71*(10), 935–963. https://doi.org/10.1002/jclp.22200

Baslet, G., Dworetzky, B., Perez, D. L., & Oser, M. (2015). Treatment of psychogenic non-epileptic seizures: Updated review and findings from a mindfulness-based intervention case series. *Clinical EEG and Neuroscience, 46*(1), 54–64. https://doi.org/10.1177/1550059414557025

Bédard, M., Felteau, M., Marshall, S., Cullen, N., Gibbons, C., Dubois, S. . . . Moustgaard, A. (2013). Mindfulness-based cognitive therapy reduces symptoms of depression in people with a traumatic brain injury: Results from a randomized controlled trial. *The Journal of Head Trauma Rehabilitation, 29*(4), E13–E22. https://doi.org/10.1097/HTR.0b013e3182a615a0

Bédard, M., Felteau, M., Marshall, S., Dubois, S., Gibbons, C., Klein, R., & Weaver, B. (2012). Mindfulness-based cognitive therapy: Benefits in reducing depression following a traumatic brain injury. *Advances in Mind-Body Medicine, 26*(1), 14–20.

Blankespoor, R. J., Schellekens, M. P. J., Vos, S. H., Speckens, A. E. M., & de Jong, B. A. (2017). The effectiveness of mindfulness-based stress reduction on psychological distress and cognitive functioning in patients with multiple sclerosis: A pilot study. *Mindfulness, 8,* 1251–1258. https://doi.org/10.1007/s12671-017-0701-6

Bogosian, A., Hughes, A., Norton, S., Silber, E., & Moss-Morris, R. (2016). Potential treatment mechanisms in a mindfulness-based intervention for people with progressive multiple sclerosis. *British Journal of Health Psychology, 21*(4), 859–880. https://doi.org/10.1111/bjhp.12201

Bowen, S., Chawla, N., & Marlatt, G. (2010). *Mindfulness-based relapse prevention for addictive behaviours: A clinician's guide*. New York: Guilford Press.

Burschka, J. M., Keune, P. M., Oy, U. H.-V., Oschmann, P., & Kuhn, P. (2014). Mindfulness-based interventions in multiple sclerosis: Beneficial effects of Tai Chi on balance, coordination, fatigue and depression. *BMC Neurology, 14*(1), 525–529. https://doi.org/10.1186/s12883-014-0165-4

Cash, T. V., Ekouevi, V. S., Kilbourn, C., & Lageman, S. K. (2016). Pilot study of a mindfulness-based group intervention for individuals with Parkinson's Disease an and their caregivers. *Mindfulness, 7*, 361–371. https://doi.org/10.1007/s12671-015-0452-1

Cavalera, C., Rovaris, M., Mendozzi, L., Pugnetti, L., Garegnani, M., Castelnuovo, G. . . . Pagnini, F. (2019). Online meditation training for people with multiple sclerosis: A randomized controlled trial. *Multiple Scerosis, 25*(4), 610–617. https://doi.org/10.1177/1352458518761187

Chen, K. W., Berger, C. C., Manheimer, E., Forde, D., Magidson, J., Dachman, L., & Lejuez, C. W. (2012). Meditative therapies for reducing anxiety: A systematic review and meta-analysis of randomized controlled trials. *Depression and Anxiety, 29*(7), 545–562. https://doi.org/10.1002/da.21964

Chiesa, A., Calati, R., & Serretti, A. (2011). Does mindfulness training improve cognitive abilities? A systematic review of neuropsychological findings. *Clinical Psychology Review, 31*(3), 449–464. https://doi.org/10.1016/j.cpr.2010.11.003

Cohen, J. (1988). *Statistical power analysis for the behavioural sciences* (2nd ed.). Hillsdale, NJ: Lawrence Erlbaum Associates.

Cresentinin, C., Matix, A., Cimenti, M., Pascoli, E., Eleopra, R., & Fabbro, F. (2018). Effect of mindfulness meditation on personality and psychological well-being in patients with multiple sclerosis. *International Journal of MS Care, 20*, 101–108.

Detert, N., & Douglass, L. (2014). Mindfulness MBSR/MBCT in a UK public health neurological service: Depression, anxiety, and perceived stress outcomes in a heterogeneous clinical sample of ninety-eight Patients with neurological or functional neurological disorders. *Neuro-Disability & Psychotherapy, 2*(1/2), 137–156.

Dickinson, J., Friary, P., & McCann, C. M. (2017). The influence of mindfulness meditation on communication and anxiety: A case study of a person with aphasia. *Aphasiology, 31*(9), 1044–1058. https://doi.org/10.1080/02687038.2016.1234582

Dissanayaka, N. N. W., Idu Jion, F., Pachana, N. A., O'Sullivan, J. D., Marsh, R., Byrne, G. J., & Harnett, P. (2016). Mindfulness for motor and nonmotor dysfunctions in Parkinson's disease. *Parkinson's Disease, 4*, 13. Article ID 7109052. https://doi.org/10.1155/2016/7109052

Edwards, M. J., Adams, R. A., Brown, H., Pareés, I., & Friston, K. J. (2012). A Bayesian account of "hysteria". *Brain, 135*(11), 3495–3512. https://doi.org/10.1093/brain/aws129

Fitzpatrick, L., Simpson, J., & Smith, A. (2010). A qualitative analysis of Mindfulness-based Cognitive Therapy (MBCT) in Parkinson's disease. *Psychology and Psychotherapy: Theory, Research and Practice, 83*(2), 179–192. https://doi.org/10.1348/147608309X471514

Frontario, A., Feld, E., Sherman, K., Krupp, L., & Charvet, L. (2016). Telehealth mindfulness meditation improves cognitive performance in adults with multiple sclerosis. *Neurology, 86*(16 Supplement), P3.092.

Gotink, R. A., Chu, P., Busschbach, J. J. V., Benson, H., Fricchione, G. L., & Hunink, M. G. M. (2015). Standardised mindfulness-based interventions in healthcare: An overview of systematic reviews and meta-analyses of RCTs. *PLoS One, 10*(4), 17. Article ID 0124344. https://doi.org/10.1371/journal.pone.0124344

Grossman, P., Kappos, L., Gensicke, H., D'Souza, M., Mohr, D. C., Penner, I. K., & Steiner, C. (2010). MS quality of life, depression, and fatigue improve after mindfulness training: A randomized trial. *Neurology, 75*(13), 1141–1149. https://doi.org/10.1212/WNL.0b013e3181f4d80d

Grossman, P., Tiefenthaler-Gilmer, U., Raysz, A., & Kesper, U. (2007). Mindfulness training as an intervention for fibromyalgia: Evidence of postintervention and 3-year follow-up benefits in well-being. *Psychotherapy and Psychosomatics, 76*(4), 226–233. https://doi.org/10.1159/000101501

Haut, S. R., Lipton, R. B., Cornes, S., Dwivedi, A. K., Wasson, R., Cotton, S. . . . Privitera, M. (2018). Behavioural interventions as a treatment for epilepsy: A multicentre randomized controlled trial. *Neurology, 90*(11). https://doi.org/10.1212/WNL.0000000000005109

Hoogerwerf, A. E. W., Bol, Y., Lobbestael, J., Hupperts, R., & Van Heugten, C. M. (2017). Mindfulness based cognitive therapy for severely fatigued multiple sclerosis patients: A waiting list controlled study. *Journal of Rehabilitation Medicine, 49*, 497–504. https://doi.org/10.2340/16501977-2237

Jensen, C. G., Vangkilde, S., Frokjaer, V., & Hasselbalch, S. G. (2012). Mindfulness training affects attention – Or is it attentional effort? *Journal of Experimental Psychology, General, 141*(1), 106–123. https://doi.org/10.1037/a0024931

Johansson, B., Bjuhr, H., & Rönnbäck, L. (2012). Mindfulness-based Stress Reduction (MBSR) improves long-term mental fatigue after stroke or traumatic brain injury. *Brain Injury, 26*(13–14), 1621–1628. https://doi.org/10.3109/02699052.2012.700082

Kolahkaj, B., & Zargar, F. (2015). Effect of mindfulness-based stress reduction on anxiety, depression and stress in women with multiple sclerosis. *Nursing and Midwifery Studies, 4*(4), 1–6. https://doi.org/10.17795/nmsjournal29655

Laures-Gore, J., & Marshall, R. S. (2016). Mindfulness meditation in aphasia: A case report. *NeuroRehabilitation, 38*, 321–329. https://doi.org/10.3233/NRE-161323

Marshall, R. S., Laures-Gore, J., & Love, K. (2018). Brief mindfulness meditation group training in aphasia: Exploring attention, language and psychophysiological outcomes. *International Journal of Language & Communication Disorders, 53*(1), 40–54. https://doi.org/10.1111/1460-6984.12325

McHugh, L., & Wood, R. (2013). Stimulus over-selectivity in temporal brain injury: Mindfulness as a potential intervention. *Brain Injury, 27*(13–14), 1595–1599. https://doi.org/10.3109/02699052.2013.834379

McMillan, T., Robertson, I. H., Brock, D., & Chorlton, L. (2002). Brief mindfulness training for attentional problems after traumatic brain injury: A randomised control treatment trial. *Neuropsychological Rehabilitation, 12*(2), 117–125.

Mills, N., & Allen, J. (2000). Mindfulness of movement as a coping strategy in multiple sclerosis: A pilot study. *General Hospital Psychiatry, 22*(6), 425–431.

Mohamadirizi, S., Shaygannejad, V., & Mohamadirizi, S. (2017). The survey of mindfulness in multiple sclerosis patients and its association with attachment style. *Journal of Education and Health Promotion, 6*(7). https://doi.org/10.4103/jehp.jehp_114_14

Nielsen, G., Stone, J., Matthews, A., Brown, M., Sparkes, C., Framer, R. . . . Edwards, M. (2015). Physiotherapy for functional motor disorders: A consensus recommendation. *Journal of Neurology, Neurosurgery and Psychiatry, 86*(10), 1113–1119. https://doi.org/10.1136/jnnp-2014-309255

Orenstein, E., Basilakos, A., & Marshall, R. S. (2012). Effects of mindfulness meditation on three individuals with aphasia. *International Journal of Language & Communication Disorders, 47*(6), 673–684. https://doi.org/10.1111/j.1460-6984.2012.00173.x

Pagnini, F., Cavalera, C., Rovaris, M., Mendozzi, L., Molinari, E., Phillips, D., & Langer, E. (2019). Longitudinal associations between mindfulness and well-being in people with multiple sclerosis. *International Journal of Clinical and Health Psychology*, *19*(1), 22–30. https://doi.org/10.1016/j.ijchp.2018.11.003

Pickut, B. A., Van Hecke, W., Kerckhofs, E., Mariën, P., Vanneste, S., Cras, P., & Parizel, P. M. (2013). Mindfulness based intervention in Parkinson's disease leads to structural brain changes on MRI: A randomized controlled longitudinal trial. *Clinical Neurology and Neurosurgery*, *115*(12), 2419–2425. https://doi.org/10.1016/j.clineuro.2013.10.002

Pickut, B. A., Vanneste, S., Hirsch, M. A., Van Hecke, W., Kerckhofs, E., Mariën, P. . . . Cras, P. (2015). Mindfulness training among individuals with Parkinson's disease: Neurobehavioral effects. *Parkinson's Disease*, *6*. Article ID 816404. https://doi.org/10.1155/2015/816404

Piet, J., & Hougaard, E. (2011). The effect of mindfulness-based cognitive therapy for prevention of relapse in recurrent major depressive disorder: A systematic review and meta-analysis. *Clinical Psychology Review*, *31*(6), 1032–1040. https://doi.org/10.1016/j.cpr.2011.05.002

Schmidt, S., Grossman, P., Schwarzer, B., Jena, S., Naumann, J., & Walach, H. (2011). Treating fibromyalgia with mindfulness-based stress reduction: Results from a 3-armed randomized controlled trial. *Pain*, *152*(2), 361–369. https://doi.org/10.1016/j.pain.2010.10.043

Schöne, B., Gruber, T., Graetz, S., Bernhof, M., & Malinowski, P. (2018). Mindful breath awareness meditation facilitates efficiency gains in brain networks: A steady-state visually evoked potentials study. *Scientific Reports*, *8*(1), 13687.

Segal, Z. V., Williams, J. M. G., & Teasdale, J. D. (2002). *Mindfulness-based cognitive therapy for depression: A new approach to preventing relapse*. New York: Guilford Press.

Segal, Z. V., Williams, J. M. G., & Teasdale, J. D. (2013). *Mindfulness-based cognitive therapy for depression* (2nd ed.). New York: Guilford Press.

Senders, A., Borgatti, A., Hanes, D., & Shonto, L. (2018). Association between pain and mindfulness in multiple sclerosis. *International Journal of MS Care*, *20*(1), 28–34. https://doi.org/10.7224/1537.2016-076

Senders, A., Bourdette, D., Hanes, D., Yadav, V., & Shinto, L. (2014). Perceived stress in multiple sclerosis: The potential role of mindfulness in health and well-being. *Journal of Evidence Based Complementary and Alternative Medicine*, *19*(4), 104–111. https://doi.org/10.1177/2156587214523291

Simpson, R. J. (2017). *Mindfulness-based interventions for people with multiple sclerosis*. Doctoral dissertation. Retrieved from Glasgow Theses Service (Unique ID glathesis:2016–7871).

Simpson, R. J., Byrne, S., Wood, K., Mair, F. S., & Mercer, S. W. (2018). Optimising mindfulness-based stress reduction for people with multiple sclerosis. *Chronic Illness*, *14*(2), 154–166. https://doi.org/10.1177/1742395317715504

Strauss, C., Cavanagh, K., Oliver, A., & Pettman, D. (2014). Mindfulness-based interventions for people diagnosed with a current episode of an anxiety or depressive disorder: A meta-analysis of randomised controlled trials. *PLoS One*, *9*(4), e96110 https://doi.org/10.1371/journal.pone.0096110

Tang, V., Poon, W. S., & Kwan, P. (2015). Mindfulness-based therapy for drug-resistant epilepsy: An assessor-blinded randomized trial. *Neurology*, *85*(13), 1100–1107. https://doi.org/10.1212/WNL.0000000000001967

Tavee, J., Rensel, M., Planchon, S. M., Butler, R. S., & Stone, L. (2011). Effects of meditation on pain and quality of life in multiple sclerosis and peripheral neuropathy. *International Journal of MS Care*, *13*, 163–168.

Thompson, N. J., Patel, A. H., Selwa, L. M., Stoll, S. C., Begley, C. E., Johnson, E. K., & Fraser, R. T. (2015). Expanding the efficacy of project UPLIFT: Distance delivery of mindfulness-based depression prevention to people with epilepsy. *Journal of Consulting and Clinical Psychology, 83*(2), 304–313. https://doi.org/10.1037/a0038404

Ulrichsen, K. M., Kaufmann, T., Dørum, E. S., Kolskår, K. K., Richard, G., Alnæs, D. . . . Nordvik, J. E. (2016). Clinical utility of mindfulness training in the treatment of fatigue after stroke, traumatic brain injury and multiple sclerosis: A systematic literature review and meta-analysis. *Frontiers in Psychology, 7*, 912. https://doi.org/10.3389.fpsyg.2016.00912

van Ravesteijn, H., Lucassen, P., Bor, H., van Weel, C., & Speckens, A. (2013). Mindfulness-based cognitive therapy for patients with medically unexplained symptoms: A randomized controlled trial. *Psychotherapy and Psychosomatics, 82*(5), 299–310. https://doi.org/10.1159/000348588

Van Vugt, M. K. (2015). Cognitive benefits of mindfulness meditation. In K. W. Brown, J. D. Cresswell, & R. M. Ryan (Eds.), *Handbook of mindfulness: Theory, research, and practice.* New York: Guilford Press.

Williams, J. M. G., Teasdale, J. D., Segal, Z. V., & Kabat-Zinn, J. (2007). *The mindful way through depression: freeing yourself from chronic unhappiness.* New York: Guilford Press.

Zigmond, A. S., & Snaith, R. P. (1983). The hospital anxiety and depression scale. *Acta Psychiatrica Scaninavica, 67*(6), 361–370.

4

WORKING WITH PEOPLE WITH ACQUIRED NEUROLOGICAL CONDITIONS AND THEIR FAMILIES

Personal construct psychology

Cathy Sparkes

This chapter aims to introduce Personal Construct Psychology (PCP) and demonstrate how its use can support, explain and enlighten professionals when working with people with acquired neurological conditions and their families and friends. PCP offers alternative ways of listening to, understanding and working creatively with individuals.

The chapter is divided into the following sections:

1   Theory, background and philosophy of PCP
2   Evidence base
3   Considerations of PCP to neurological conditions
4   Suitability
5   Case example: Dom
6   Practitioner's reflections on using PCP with neurological conditions

Theory, background and philosophy of PCP

PCP is a theory developed by George Kelly in 1955. It is a comprehensive theory of personality and applies to everyone. Six key aspects of the theory are:

1   Philosophy
2   Constructs and construing
3   Person-the-scientist
4   Dependency
5   Credulous approach
6   Reflexivity

Philosophy

Kelly (1955/1991) says 'We take the stand that there are always some alternative constructions available to choose among in dealing with the world'. He goes on to say that we need never paint ourselves into a corner nor be completely hemmed in by circumstances and that no-one needs to be 'the victim of their biography'. Kelly calls this philosophical position 'Constructive Alternativism'. He was keen to ensure that his theory was embedded in the wider context of someone's way of interacting with the world. He suggests that each individual is trying to grasp the real world but can only construct their own version of it. The construction that someone can make of the world is infinitely variable. Kelly's underlying notions of alternatives and choice are key for a client and practitioner to take on board as they work together to open up the options the client has and that they both have within therapy.

Constructs and construing

PCP proposes that each of us sees the world through unique transparent patterns or templates that we create and then attempt 'to fit over the realities of which the world is composed' (Kelly, 1955/1991). Kelly suggests that construing (the act of making sense of the world) and developing one's own personal 'construct system' starts before birth and continues throughout a person's life, gradually becoming more elaborate and defined. Infants are construing even before they have access to words (pre-verbal), for example through their sense of mother rather than not-mother, or hungry rather than satisfied. As language and cognition changes through childhood, adolescence and onto adulthood, a person's construing continues to develop at both nonverbal and verbal levels. Each person's construct system is affected and shaped by interactions, experiences, contexts and culture through all our senses and behaviours. An individual will use their own personal construct system as a way to help anticipate, predict and exert control over what might and can happen in the future.

Constructs are bi-polar discriminations of similarities and differences between elements such as people, objects and events. The nature between the two poles of a construct is one of contrast. When an individual construes something in a certain way, that person is implicitly stating what it is not to them. Examples of constructs include large rather than small, trapped rather than free, tidy rather than disorganised. Everyone's construing is different, so whilst one person might have a construct 'tidy' rather than 'disorganised', another may have 'tidy' rather than 'obsessive'.

An individual's construct system is a multidimensional, interconnected, flexible structure which consists of a vast number of constructs that are variously linked to each other. Constructs occur:

- at different levels of awareness (pre-verbal, nonverbal and verbal);
- in a hierarchy from superordinate (more overarching and abstract) to subordinate (relating more to tangible behaviours);

- with differing degrees of importance – from core constructs (important and less open to change) to peripheral constructs (less important and more open to change).

The role of the practitioner is to investigate and understand the construct system of the client in order to form the basis for therapy and intervention. This could be structured like the Repertory Grid (Kelly, 1955/1991), however most practitioners take a more informal and conversational approach.

Person-the-scientist

Kelly (1955/1991) proposes that everyone is in their 'own particular way, a scientist'. Behaviour is seen as an experiment to test out our theory of the world. In everyday life everyone conducts 'experiments' (intentionally or unintentionally, small or large) to test out their current perceptions, interpretations and constructions of the world. Each person develops a hypothesis, experiments through their behaviour and becomes aware of the consequences. If the outcome of an experiment is as predicted then the behaviour and experiment is 'validated', and an individual may continue on that path. However, if an outcome is not as predicted or 'invalidated', an individual may seek to understand why or how the experiment did not give rise to the predicted outcome. Neither outcome is positive or negative, but both are an opportunity to learn about oneself. A practitioner working with an individual in this way can support the person's self-understanding and facilitate further hypotheses and experimentation. Through this process, personal reconstructions may take place and different behaviours can be experimented with.

Dependency

Rather than aiming for independence, PCP encourages us to explore the concept of dependence, by spreading our needs widely, in differentiated ways and recognising whom to turn to for what. In fact Dalton (2005) asserts: 'PCP argues that dependence is both necessary and desirable'. PCP proposes that people can thrive when they have access to a range of people and resources at different times and in diverse ways. If an individual relies heavily on only one or two people, problems may arise if these relationships come under strain. Equally if someone spreads their dependence in an overly dispersed way this too can be unhelpful, overly diluted and in some ways superficial. Working with a client within their social relationships in an experimental way can help them to understand how and why they might and can depend on others. This concept applies to family members and friends too, who might need support to find a range of useful and appropriate people and services to turn to as they manage their new relationship dynamics with each other. Likewise, a practitioner might find it helpful to turn to one person for supervision, an organisation for support, a specialist for mentoring and a peer for collaboration. Kelly (1955/1991) maintains: 'The task of therapy is to enable the client to differentiate between his dependencies, to wrap them up in small packages so that they may be appropriately allocated and distributed among different people'.

Credulous approach

Through the practitioner openly listening to and not making assumptions about the story a client tells, their relationship grows and develops. As Fransella and Dalton (1990) write, 'If the ability to suspend one's own and subsume another's construing system are vital skills a personal construct counsellor must possess, then the ability to listen credulously is the first stage of "getting into" the client's system'. The practitioner attempts to step into the shoes of that individual and in PCP terms offers a 'credulous approach'. This requires the practitioner to suspend their own construing as far as possible and subsume (see the world through the eyes of) the construing of the client. These skills are at the heart of a PCP approach, which encourages the practitioner to gain a thorough understanding of the client's construing in order to develop hypotheses regarding how they are experiencing their difficulties and in turn develop useful opportunities for experimentation.

Reflexivity

Fransella (2005) highlights that in all our interactions, the same explanatory framework is equally applicable to both parties – to scientist and subject, therapist and client, husband and wife and parent and child. PCP reminds the practitioner to observe not only the construing, responses and behaviours of each client but also to reflect on their own constructs, patterns of construing and opportunities for experimentation. This is what is understood by the term 'reflexivity' within PCP.

Evidence base

PCP has been applied to many domains, including clinical, educational and organisational fields, and a body of research has developed. Walker and Winter (2007) suggest, 'The extent of the subsequent fit in extremely diverse fields may be far greater than even Kelly could have anticipated'. Watson and Winter (2005) reflect that Personal Construct Therapy is under-researched, but their process and outcome study provided considerable evidence for the effectiveness of personal construct psychotherapy with diagnostically heterogeneous clients. Their study demonstrated that it is possible to carry out a study of process and outcome in personal construct therapy in a real setting with clients who are representative of those typically seen in practice.

Winter (2003) summarises that there is a growing body of evidence that indicates that:

- psychological disorders are characterised by particular features of construing;
- effective psychological therapy is associated with reconstruing;

- the process of personal construct psychotherapy is distinctive and contrasts in practice with that in rationalist cognitive therapy;
- personal construct psychotherapy is effective, in an individual or group format, with a range of client groups;
- The degree of improvement in this form of therapy is similar to that in other therapies.

Winter (2003) provides us with a comprehensive summary of clinical research that has been carried out looking at the use of PCP in a wide range of clients, groups and settings. He reflects that much of the research in the field of PCP has been through the use of Repertory Grid technique (Kelly, 1955/1991), a structured approach that examines how a client uses their constructs in relation to a set of elements (typically people). The client's constructs can be mapped onto and represented on a structured grid. In the neurological field, Brumfitt (1985) used this method with people with restricted communication following a stroke. Elements used included past self, self when struggling to talk now, self when not talking now, ideal self, spouse, child/brother/sister, someone you feel sorry for and a friend. Due to their language difficulties, photographs were used as a way to facilitate the dialogue and elicit the constructs for each client. Brumfitt concludes that the use of a grid can be of benefit to understand the construct system of a client with a neurological condition and communication difficulties, for the client themselves to understand their own constructs and to recognise that construing occurs in the absence of language. Brumfitt (2000) goes on to explain that in addition to the grid, other methods, for example self-characterisation (Kelly, 1955/1991), which is a self-description written in the third person, can provide theoretical insights for the practitioner and client following a stroke.

Gracey et al. (2008) used PCP and qualitative research to investigate how people construe themselves after brain injury. They concluded that 'following brain injury people make sense of themselves in terms of the meanings and felt experiences of social and practical activity'. More recently, in the field of acquired brain injury, Coppock (2017) carried out a study looking at three families where one parent within each has experienced an acquired brain injury. Coppock asserts that the application of PCP theory can provide a framework for understanding individual and family experiences that could help facilitate therapeutic support and suggests that practitioners might benefit from listening credulously to enable the identification of each family's unique needs. These recent investigations have offered some helpful insights into the benefits of PCP within this client group.

Considerations of PCP to neurological conditions

Each individual will try to use their personal knowledge and personal constructs to help predict and control their world. However, many individuals with a neurological condition will be unable to rely on past knowledge, behaviours or personal constructs as they once were able to. Someone with a neurological condition may present with an array of difficulties that could impact their own sense of identity, their ability to form and maintain relationships and their capacity to anticipate the future. Clients typically want to work towards how and who they used to be. The role of the practitioner is to assist the client to determine those aspects of their past identity and construing that remain relevant and which aspects may require reconstruction.

Four PCP approaches which may support people with neurological conditions along with those in their support network are described here:

1   Getting to know someone: Constructs and creativity
2   Building relationships: Using a credulous approach
3   Testing out new ways of being: Person-the-scientist
4   Clients in context: Spreading dependence

Getting to know someone: Constructs and creativity

In each therapy session, the practitioner strives to create a safe space to allow the client to share how they are construing what has happened, what is happening and their anticipations for the future. The practitioner aims to create the opportunity for conversations about a client's expectations from therapy, their hopes for the outcomes of intervention and the purpose of their work together. Expectations and hopes (for life and therapy) will depend on the client's personal constructs around areas in which they may or may not have had previous experience. These might include unexpected change, therapy, help, dependence, disability and living with difference. Dalton (2005) reflects how Kelly 'sees therapist and client as partners in the enterprise, each having their own area of expertise'. Fundamental to this partnership is a cooperative relationship where the client comes to recognise and believe that they are the authority on themselves, from before the start of their condition, in the present and going forward. Meanwhile the practitioner is an expert in helping the client to explore their concerns, offering alternative perspectives and helping to set up experiments for change.

It is the practitioner's role to address in what ways a client's construing can support them in their new situation, to understand how their current construing may be a barrier to progress and in what ways they can move forward. As clients may have cognitive and communication difficulties, the introduction of practical and creative resources can serve a useful purpose. Many clients with neurological conditions struggle to access words, ideas and concepts around their experience. However, sometimes taking a sensory route (visual, tactile) to someone's personal constructs can open up otherwise difficult interactions. Materials can include those in the client's immediate context (items on their person or in the room) and/or those brought by the practitioner (paper and pens, postcards, photos or three-dimensional materials such as buttons, shells and stones). Through using a combination of creative resources, each client has opportunities to express who they were, who they are now and what is important to them going forward. PCP can help provide ways not only to explore and understand a client's construct system but also to enable a practitioner to become aware of and recognise their own construing in relation to that client (reflexivity).

Building relationships: Using a credulous approach

PCP is a conversation-based approach with techniques and tools that can be used flexibly to support the therapeutic process. There is no set schedule or format to follow to subsume each client's construing. Building a respectful relationship with a client is important in the exploration of pre-existing personal constructs and possible areas of change. Working credulously with this particular client group can be demanding, as many such clients have difficulties in areas of self-awareness and insight, creating potential barriers to moving forward productively. A practitioner may see a client whose cognitive difficulties are affecting their behaviour. But these behaviours may also relate to their need to hold tightly to their core constructs such as 'working' rather than 'unemployed', 'strong and capable' rather than 'weak and needing help'.

The client and practitioner must explore together the client's new world and aim to determine what impact the client's construing has on their way of living and behaving. To gain access to a client's construing, one useful technique is 'Self-characterisation' (Kelly, 1955/1991). This is an opportunity for a client to write about (or in other ways represent) themselves in the third person, as if standing in the shoes of someone else. This process and the subsequent reflections by the client and practitioner can open an extremely rich and fertile exchange and assist the practitioner in stepping into the world of the client. Through taking a credulous approach, the practitioner begins to understand how the client's behaviour may relate to their construing of a situation or barrier rather than the situation or barrier itself.

Testing out new ways of being: Person-the-scientist

The idea of 'person-the-scientist' can readily apply to clients with neurological conditions in their 'new' life and can allow an individual to test out their construing and behaviours. The client and practitioner set up experiments together so that the client can return to a further session with their experience or particular 'data' to review. For example, Robert wanted to be 'outgoing' again. He had always construed himself as an *outgoing* rather than a *reserved* individual. His neurological condition resulted in problems with talking, tiredness and feeling low. The practitioner helped Robert to choose areas to explore, set up useful experiments to enable him to determine if he could still be *outgoing*, as he now construed it, across a range of activities and situations. They then reviewed those experiments to see if his hypotheses had been validated or invalidated. With either outcome, the process enabled reflection of what happened and discussion around changes that Robert recognised needed to be made as a result.

Robert started his experiments with situations which were less daunting and then progressed to ones which were more so:

• Attending a local group for people with aphasia (including sessions playing golf and cycling): experiment validated. He still attends.

- Taking a trip to London on his own: experiment validated. He continues to take trips and has increased their frequency.
- Attending an aphasia 'drop in' group in London: experiment validated. Robert felt he behaved in a 'confident' and 'outgoing' way and received feedback from others in the group to that effect. He still attends.
- Assisting in lectures (speaking in small groups and to a larger audience) at a university for SLT students: experiment validated.
- Returning to work for three months in a different role: experiment invalidated. Robert was unable to be 'outgoing' in the work context due to his communication difficulties.

As a result of these experiments, Robert construes himself again as 'outgoing' in social situations. Offering the idea of person-the-scientist and setting up meaningful experiments with feedback is a fundamental pillar within PCP as a means of facilitating change.

Clients in context: Spreading dependence

An individual client with a neurological condition can often find themselves in a situation where they are depending for help and support on very few people (partner, parent, neighbour, therapist, GP). PCP can help an individual notice whether their support network has remained constant or if it has altered. A practitioner and client might work towards increasing the breadth of people and services the client can turn to and to understand how to differentiate between those elements. Hopefully the client will become more aware of who they are turning to for what and how their dependencies might affect relationships over time. The practitioner can help suggest people to experiment with, and the client can test out their new constructions. This could range from one or more individuals, to groups, events and organisations. Key for the client and family to understand, is the value of a spread of dependence and the discrimination between different sources of support.

Suitability

Here, rather than considering whom the approach is suitable for, since it is widely acknowledged as being suitable for everyone, it might be more relevant to ask: In what ways can PCP theory be used in relation to those we are working with or alongside?

Dalton (2005) reflects that:

> PCP does not bring any ready-made model of the meaning of 'symptoms' to work with clients. With the essential focus on the person's *own* meanings, therapist and client explore the ways in which these views themselves might be keeping the person unable to change things for the better.

PCP can help the practitioner understand their own and others' construing and thereby inform their approach with all client groups. As a theory for everyone, a PCP approach can inform the basis for involvement with any client including introductory sessions, one-off consultations, regular sessions, family interventions, longer term ongoing support or periodic reviews.

A PCP approach offers the practitioner and the client:

- ways to understand how the client construes themselves and the world around them;
- an understanding of the client's constructs with respect to the timing and nature of therapeutic intervention;
- a peer dialogue where the client can have a say in and take responsibility for determining what works for them;
- a variety of approaches to help the client increase their understanding of how their own constructs are being affected by an event or situation;
- flexible and creative means by which the client can express their constructs when there are cognitive and/or communication difficulties;
- a platform to explore alternatives relating to the client's relationships, how they are addressing questions, concerns and dilemmas, and their future possibilities when facing very limited life choices;
- the opportunity to set up a range of relevant and useful experiments to help the client understand their own choices and make life more meaningful in relation to their present circumstances;
- the freedom to explore alternative therapeutic approaches which can be accessed instead of or alongside a PCP approach;
- regular reviews, at suitable intervals as appropriate, in order to create space for the client to evaluate the effectiveness of experiments conducted or the approaches being offered.

Case example: Dom

Dom had a stroke at 29; he is now 42. He had a job, a girlfriend and a bright future. Five years after his stroke, Dom was referred for counselling. At that time, he was living in his own property with live-in carers. Dom reported that his self-esteem was extremely low as he felt trapped by multiple disabilities (physical, cognitive and communication), a variety of unhelpful relationships and a constant undercurrent of fatigue. He viewed his future as bleak. In contrast to Dom's upbeat exterior was an internal world in which he was struggling with a change to his identity. Dom now reflects 'My first priority was and is to work out a plan as to how to survive'.

At our first session, Dom said he wanted to take the power back in his life, and this has been a major theme throughout therapy. Dom reflects that 'no control was awful, as opposed to some control which still feels pretty awful but I am coming to terms with the fact that I do need to rely on others to do everything'.

This is an example of a core personal construct of Dom's: 'No control' rather than 'some control and relying on others'. Offering a credulous approach, I helped Dom discover how to find some control both within therapy and in his life. 'Therapy was about me – you wanted my perspective on things, you helped me with problem-solving and you validated my decision-making'.

At the start of our work together, Dom identified two main areas that he wanted to work on: 'Making living bearable' and 'Finding a girlfriend'. Both of these centred on relationships – Dom recognised that he needed to work on 'Making sure I have the right people around me'. I encouraged Dom to widen and strengthen his networks not only with people with disabilities, carers and healthcare professionals but also with old and new friends outside the community of those with a neurological condition. As a result of Dom spreading his dependence, he expanded his weekly schedule to include a mixture of concerts, gigs, having friends to visit and specific time alone. 'Good job this happened to me as I have a get up and go that others don't have. I use that to stay in touch with people. I have never been the sort of person to sit around'. Dom's construct – 'get up and go' rather than 'sitting around' – was explored, as this was a pre-stroke construct, but it was related to a physical 'get up and go'. Now he has had to reconstrue 'get up and go' as a way to motivate himself and others through communicating often via social media. Dom expressed that 'My anti-depressants are gigs' – planning them, anticipating them, meeting up with friends and posting pictures and videos on Facebook, with resulting comments and likes.

When Dom and I started to work together he knew a lot of people, but he was depending on his close family (parents and brother) and a few very specific people (whom he had not selected) for a limited number of activities. He was unsure which friends he could trust and saw many as controlling his life. He had a personal construct of 'trustworthy' as a contrast to 'controlling'. As therapy continued, Dom started to shift his distribution of dependence. Dom reflects that he has become more 'autonomous' in his life, and by that he means he can choose whom to turn to for what. He sees this now as a contrast to 'independent', which relates to relying solely on himself. Our conversations explored how Dom could balance his focus around finding a girlfriend with developing relationships with a variety of people. 'Working with you has helped me to build relationships and to help me regulate those relationships'. After two years of working together Dom reported, 'I have put finding a girlfriend on the back burner'. As more of a priority Dom realised his 'need to learn how to have a friend living here (at his house) as a carer', which became a focus within sessions.

Thirteen years after his stroke, Dom's original overarching aim of working out how to survive has changed. He has identified that his key aspirations now are twofold: 'finding reliable people in my community who I can turn to' and 'to begin to feel free in spite of my difficulties'. Together, we have focused on the circumstances in which Dom can try to put his disabilities further in the background and feel a sense of freedom, for even brief periods. My work with Dom has been a constantly evolving balancing act between credulous listening and embracing his reality. Sessions are always directed by him, and, if unsure about the next step, I would remind myself of Kelly (1955/1991): 'if you don't know what is wrong with someone, ask them, they may tell you'.

We have worked together, with our differing but complementary expertise, to enable Dom to choose those interventions within therapy and people in his life who are of most help in reconstruing his life and reconstructing his identity.

In his therapy, Dom experimented with and chose:

- a range of roles for me to play: advocate, ally, challenger, counsellor, friend, mentor, negotiator, facilitator, navigator;
- the frequency of sessions: weekly, every other week, monthly, 'as and when';
- the style and location of therapy: individual, group, with others in his network, in his house and in the community.

In his life, Dom experimented with and progressed from:

- being in an unstable and difficult living arrangement through to one where he has greater choice and security;
- feeling confined in his own home through to an active social life and travelling abroad;
- accessing intensive but unhelpful therapy through to securing a personally selected and beneficial configuration of support;
- overreliance on his parents through to turning to a wider community and network of family and friends who can help him with short-term needs and longer-term plans.

Practitioner's reflections on using PCP with neurological conditions

I started as a Speech and Language Therapist (SLT) in 1986 and worked with people with a range of neurological conditions in a number of different NHS settings. My specific interest has always been neurorehabilitation, and I have worked with a wide variety of clients, families and multidisciplinary team colleagues. After I qualified as an SLT, I soon realised that although fascinated by communication, I was equally if not more intrigued by the person. In 1988, I attended a PCP Foundation Course run by Peggy Dalton, who worked as an SLT and psychotherapist, specialising in working with people with neurological conditions and those who stammer. She also had personal experience of living with someone with a neurological condition, which gave her a unique perspective on her clinical work and in turn my own practice. From her professional and personal experiences, Dalton (1990) reflected that the most important thing anyone can do for someone who has experienced a devastating loss is to accept and respect what is meaningful for them − to be truly credulous about their experience.

I was particularly drawn to PCP, as it acknowledges that we are all individuals who are trying to make sense of, understand and construe the world around us. The PCP Foundation Course changed my practice and my life. I studied and qualified as a PCP Counsellor and Psychotherapist (2003) and since then have worked as an independent PCP Practitioner including the roles of counsellor, supervisor and coach. My dual training (as SLT and counsellor) has taken me into varied contexts including charitable organisations, higher education establishments and multiprofessional forums. In my work, I continue to apply the theory to individuals, to groups and of course to myself.

Whilst PCP is a theoretical structure that enables me to understand, describe and develop the way a person makes sense of events, it is also a practical and innovative way to design appropriate and effective intervention for individuals, including those who have disabilities resulting from a neurological condition. My own experience and experimentation with this theory is an important feature of why I believe it works. I consider that my interest and faith in it has made a significant difference to the outcomes of my work with and alongside clients, families and colleagues.

PCP is a springboard for helping me to understand how I and others see the world and how therapy might play a positive part in changing an individual's way of construing the world. I have embraced and utilised it for over 30 years now, both in times of calm and moments of conflict. It has provided me with the tools to think creatively about people and situations. I find PCP a constructive and accepting theory. It provides a strong but flexible structure that enables me to work with people who are complex and vulnerable, and it helps me to see the individual differences in clients. The theory and practice provide a way of enhancing my already strong commitment to encouraging personal development and realising potential. PCP provides and sustains my optimism and belief that there are always choices for people. The individual may or may not be able to recognise those choices, accept them or work with them. However, working together, the client and the practitioner can both actively explore choices, experiment and reconstrue their views of their world, often for the better.

To conclude this chapter, I invited Dom to say some final words about our work together.

> When we first met I had no control in my life but people controlling it. Piece by piece you have helped me to get a bit more control . . . the key to a good therapist is always to be able to get on with them, look forward to seeing them and have a laugh. You have helped me with my thoughts, listened to my moaning and understood that I am often tired and depressed. Most of all, though, you have validated an in-valid life and by that I mean someone who is unsure about what they are doing. You did not offer me advice but have pointed me towards things. You have always come prepared for sessions with me but often it's that you are equipped to listen to me talk about absolutely anything.

Thanks to Mary Frances for her inspiration, Helen Jones for her wisdom, Deborah Harding for her support and Woody for his tolerance and attention to detail.

References

Brumfitt, S. (1985). The use of repertory grids with aphasic people. In N. Beail (Ed.), *Repertory grid technique and personal constructs.* London: Croom Helm.

Brumfitt, S. (2000). Personal construct theory in stroke and communication problems. In R. Fawcus (Ed.), *Stroke rehabilitation: A collaborative approach.* New Jersey: Wiley-Blackwell.

Coppock, C., Winter, D., Ferguson, S., & Green, A. (2017). Using the Perceiver Element Grid (PEG) to elicit intrafamily construal following parental acquired brain injury. *Personal Construct Theory & Practice, 14,* 25–39.

Dalton, P. (1990). *Living in the present: The experience of amnesia.* Paper presented at the Second British Conference on PCP, College of Ripon and York St. John.

Dalton, P., & Dunnett, G. (2005). *A psychology for living: Personal construct theory for professionals and clients* (2nd ed.). New Jersey: Wiley-Blackwell.

Fransella, F. (Ed.). (2005). *The essential practitioners handbook of personal construct psychology.* New Jersey: Wiley-Blackwell.

Fransella, F., & Dalton, P. (1990). *Personal construct counselling in action.* London: Sage Publications.

Gracey, F., Palmer, S., Rous, B., Psaila, K., Shaw, K., O'Dell, J., Mohamed, S. (2008). "Feeling part of things": Personal construction of self after brain injury. *Neuropsychological Rehabilitation, 18*(5–6), 627–650.

Kelly, G. (1955/1991). *The psychology of personal constructs* (Volume 1: Theory and personality; Volume 2: Clinical diagnosis and psychotherapy). New York: Norton. Reprinted, London: Routledge.

Syder, D. (Ed.). (1998). *Wanting to talk: Counselling case studies in communication disorders.* London: Whurr Publishers Ltd.

Walker, B., & Winter, D. A. (2007). The elaboration of personal construct psychology. *Annual Review of Psychology, 58,* 453–477.

Watson, S., & Winter, D. A. (2005). A process and outcome study of personal construct psychotherapy. In D. A. Winter & L. L. Viney (Eds.), *Personal construct psychotherapy: Advances in theory, practice and research.* London: Whurr Publishers Ltd.

Winter, D. A. (2003). The evidence base for personal construct psychotherapy. In F. Fransella (Ed.), *International handbook of personal construct psychology* (pp. 265–272). London: Wiley-Blackwell.

5

COMPASSION FOCUSED THERAPY FOR NEUROLOGICAL CONDITIONS

Fiona Ashworth and Clara Murray

We are no strangers to suffering, in ourselves or others. We often hear the phrases 's/he suffered a brain injury' or 's/he is suffering with multiple sclerosis'. When we take a moment to think about this, to put ourselves in our clients' shoes (and their families), we can only begin to imagine the extent, the depth and the gravity of this suffering – perhaps a loss of core memories of family occasions, a loss of recognition of those nearest and dearest, a loss of a job that they loved or a hobby they were passionate about due to cognitive and physical changes or perhaps a loss of key relationships due to psychological distress or difficulties with communication. More often than not, our clients experience many of these difficulties as a result of their neurological condition (NC). The key aim of Compassion Focused Therapy (CFT) is to support clients to develop a more compassionate relationship with themselves and others in light of their suffering. Within CFT, we work from the Dalai Llama's definition that of compassion as a sensitivity to the suffering of the self and others with a deep wish and commitment to relieve that suffering.

Theory, background and philosophy of the therapy

CFT is an integrated biopsychosocial and multimodal approach to psychotherapy that draws from evolutionary, Buddhist, developmental and social psychology and neuroscience. CFT was initially developed by Professor Paul Gilbert to work with those with pervasive self-criticism and shame. Shame and self-criticism are viewed as internal experiences that can often underpin and maintain a multitude of mental health problems including depression, anxiety, eating disorders, Post-Traumatic Stress Disorder (PTSD) and personality disorders, thus they are viewed as transdiagnostic problems. There is also evidence that self-criticism and shame can be pervasive experiences for those with neurological conditions and are associated with significant psychological distress (e.g., see Ashworth, Clarke, Jones, Jennings, & Longworth, 2015). People who are highly self-critical and shamed can struggle to feel safe, reassured and soothed. One of the key aims of CFT is to help people develop and work with experiences of inner warmth, safeness and soothing, via compassion and self-compassion (Gilbert, 2009). Described here are the key principles and philosophy from which CFT is drawn.

CFT combines emphases on social psychology, positive psychology, evolutionary theory and neurophysiological models of affect regulation to understand our emotional experiences (Gilbert, 2005, 2009, 2010a, 2010b). The CFT approach argues that attachment and affiliative behaviours have evolved over hundreds of thousands of years to regulate threat-based emotions and action tendencies. For example, when children are threatened, the kindness and affection of the parent calms them down because their brains are set up to be calmed by the compassion and kindness of others. This is an important evolutionary role of affiliation and attachment, which is key to CFT. CFT focuses on developing affiliative emotions (e.g., care, support, kindness, validation and encouragement) as part of the experience of these interventions. It is the 'emotional textures' of the intervention that are key. Core to CFT is the view that our relationships with ourselves can be helpful, kind, compassionate, understanding and validating, or we can become self-critical and self-undermining. Indeed, people high in self-criticism can experience mental health issues such as anxiety and depression whereas those who are self-compassionate are more resilient (MacBeth & Gumley, 2012). Hence, one simple approach of CFT is to identify self-criticism and help people refocus on self-compassion.

CFT suggests that the way we think and feel about ourselves and others is linked to three affect regulation systems, each serving an important survival function from an evolutionary perspective. The 'three circles model' is a heuristic used in CFT to conceptualise the interplay between these systems (Gilbert, 2009). The model draws on neuroscience research on emotion by Depue and Morrone-Strupinsky (2005) and LeDoux (1998). The first affect regulation system is the threat system, which evolved to detect threat and instigate defensive/protective actions. It is associated with defensive emotions such as anger and anxiety and defensive behaviours such as fight, flight, submit and freeze responses. The threat system narrows attention and can focus rumination on threat. The neurophysiology of the threat system, and how it regulates emotional, cognitive and behavioural processes, is increasingly well understood (LeDoux, 1998). The second major affect regulating system focuses on acquiring and achieving resources. All living things need to be motivated to secure the resources required for their survival and reproduction. This system is especially associated with dopaminergic drive and motivational systems, which are energising. The third affect regulation system is linked to contentment and being neither threatened nor driven to succeed. These states are associated with quiescence. Fundamental to CFT is research that shows that this system is linked to feelings of a sense of 'peaceful wellbeing' and is often referred to as the soothing-contentment system (Carter, 1998; MacDonald & MacDonald, 2010). This system seems to be particularly involved in the attachment/affiliative system and is partly regulated through endorphins and oxytocin. Oxytocin is a hormone released by the pituitary gland associated with social behaviour and feelings of contentment. It has a direct influence on the amygdala and is associated with threat reduction (Kirsch et al., 2005).

Central to the CFT approach is the idea that the three emotion-regulation systems can be activated by both external and internal cues. The threat system can be activated by experiencing criticism or hostility from others or by being self-critical or ruminating on one's own failings or difficulties. Similarly, the CFT approach proposes that the soothing-contentment system can be activated in various ways, by actions of others or via practiced imagery, especially if it is affiliative and compassion focused. If people are kind, understanding and validating, this can help to calm and increase a sense of feeling valued and wanted. By learning to be kind, understanding and validating to ourselves, especially when struggling with difficulties, this directs us to the self-compassion process and reduces threat processing. The evolutionary focus of CFT also takes into account how much of what goes on in our minds is 'not our fault', thus working towards de-shaming the client. In addition to this, the evolutionary perspective highlights how we are all in the same boat; we all suffer, and we are part of a genetic lottery; we did not choose our genes nor the families that we were born into, and this is *not our fault*.

Underpinning CFT is Gilbert and Miles's (2000) social rank theory (SRT), which states that the way we experience our emotions is significantly affected by how we position ourselves in relation to others, e.g., superior, inferior, equal. The developmental context of an individual prior to their NC should consider how the person positions themselves in relation to others. Feeling inferior can lead to feelings of shame and self-criticism. Following a brain injury or development of a neurological condition, individuals can perceive threats (e.g., 'People look down on me') arising from the consequences of the condition, which can lead to unhelpful responses, e.g., avoidance as a coping strategy (Riley, Brennan, & Powell, 2004). Emerging studies highlight that shame and self-criticism can form part of the emotional experience following an acquired brain injury (ABI), such as a stroke or Traumatic Brain Injury (TBI), resulting in significant psychological distress (Jones & Morris, 2013; Hagger, 2011; Freeman, Adams, & Ashworth, 2015). A central theme in the experience and impact of neurological conditions is that failures or perceived failures can be experienced as threats to an individual's sense of identity, which can result in a negative sense of self (Gracey & Ownworth, 2011). It is hypothesised that following onset of their condition, some individuals may have to give up part of or all of their professional and personal social groups, which can threaten their sense of identity (Haslam et al., 2008). SRT posits that such experiences result in shame and self-criticism, e.g., 'I'm too thick to do that job now', or 'I am no longer any good at that anymore so I am a waste of space' (Gilbert & Allan, 1998). Importantly, how the person positioned themselves in relation to others prior to the ABI may exacerbate or ameliorate such difficulties.

Key components of the therapy

There are five key components to the practice of CFT (Gilbert, 2014). These are not necessarily linear and starting where the client is at in their psychological process is important. CFT differentiates between the therapy itself, which involves the therapeutic relationship, the basic concepts (psycho-education) and formulation processes, and the specific training in compassion with the individual, often referred to as Compassionate Mind Training (CMT).

1   *Psycho-education.* This component focuses on de-shaming and depersonalising through helping the client to understand the 'trickiness' of our evolved brain. The client is supported to realise that a lot of what goes on in our mind and life is 'not our fault'. The three circles model is also discussed and explored in the client's context.

2   *Formulation.* This process focuses on enabling the client to learn about how their early life experiences lead to the creation of internal strategies (how we relate within ourselves and with our emotional experiences) and external strategies (how we relate to others based on what we think is going on in their minds) for defending against threats. This also includes drive/excitement based and affiliative soothing abilities and strategies. The formulation focuses on historical context, the key fears that may have arisen as a result of this, the protective/defensive strategies used to defend against these key fears as well as the unintended consequences of these defences.

3   *Cultivating and building compassionate capacities.* This initial phase focuses on working with affiliative emotions and learning to practice parasympathetic activation via breathing exercises (e.g., soothing rhythm breathing) and imagery exercises (e.g., safe place exercise) from CMT. Initially this will also focus on building awareness of attention and learning to be mindful.

4   *Building compassionate capacity around the sense of identity.* This forms a central part of building self-compassion through behavioural practices using the compassionate-self exercise. The client will focus on learning how to take a compassionate perspective, exploring what works for them and reflecting on what they want to cultivate in the therapy.

5   *Using compassionate capacity to engage with difficulties.* Once these compassionate capacities have been developed enough, the client can be supported to use their 'compassionate mind' to engage with and work with the specific problems they are facing, for example trauma related issues, anxiety, self-criticism, depression or grief.

Evidence base for CFT

Evidence is growing for the utility of CFT in learning to cope with chronic mental health problems by training to be compassionate towards the self. Compassion based interventions have been shown to be effective for people high in self-criticism and shame, including those with anxiety, depression, eating disorders and PTSD (see Leaviss & Uttley, 2015 and Kirby, 2017 for reviews). Research has also focused on the role that compassion plays in positive mental wellbeing and highlighting that self-compassion is a protective factor for psychopathology (MacBeth & Gumley, 2012). There is emerging research to suggest that the benefits of being compassionate go above and beyond mental health and extend into developing more positive and supportive relationships with others (Neff & Beretvas, 2013; Yarnell & Neff, 2013). This is an especially important aspect for people with neurological conditions who can often find themselves isolated, and even more so if they are struggling with mental health problems.

Given the chronic and complex consequences of neurological conditions, it is unsurprising that many individuals often live in a world where they experience constant internal and external threat in the form of criticism or disappointment. This in turn can have a negative impact on their quality of life. The specific application of CFT to the treatment of neurological conditions is relatively novel within the last decade (see Ashworth, Evans, & McLeod, 2017 for a review); to date there is a combined one to one and group CFT based study following ABI (Ashworth et al., 2015), a feasibility randomised controlled trial of a CFT group for dementia (Craig, Hiskey, Royan, Poz, & Spector, 2018) and five individual case studies describing CFT in the context of neurological conditions in clinical settings (Ashworth, Gracey, & Gilbert, 2011; Shields & Ownsworth, 2013; Ashworth, 2014; Poz, 2014; Shravat, 2014). Two of the case studies, one male and one female, using CFT following a TBI report clinically significant reductions in psychological distress for both clients (Ashworth et al., 2011; Ashworth, 2014). Shravat (2014) describes the use of yoga to enhance a CFT intervention for a woman who had suffered a stroke, with qualitative reports of reduced threat activation and increased self-soothing. Poz's (2014) case study reported the usefulness of using CFT in the context of diagnosis of dementia for both the patient and partner. Shields and Ownsworth's (2013) case demonstrated a significant reduction in emotional distress and avoidant behaviours as well as an increase in self-compassion for a stroke survivor struggling to come to terms with the stroke and its consequences. The outcomes reported in the Ashworth et al. (2015) study of a range of people with ABI (N = 12) indicate significant reductions in self-criticism, anxiety and depression and a significant increase in the ability to self-reassure, i.e., the ability to soothe the self when things go wrong; a part of being self-compassionate. The data from the Craig et al. (2018) study showed improvements in mood, anxiety and self-compassion as well as three of the six participants moving out of the clinical range for depression. These initial studies have explored CFT with a variety of neurological conditions, including stroke, TBI, encephalitis, anoxic damage, post tumour neurological surgery and dementia. There are a further two experimental studies investigating brief Compassion Focused Imagery (CFI) (namely safe place imagery) for empathy deficits following TBI (O'Neill & McMillan, 2012) and brief CFI for psychological distress following TBI (Campbell, Gallagher, McLeod, O'Neill, & McMillan, 2019) with neither finding any significant changes. However there is little written about the application of CFT for other neurological conditions, and its' application needs further investigation in terms of effectiveness and adaptability. Overall, the findings to date indicate that CFT shows promise as an intervention to manage the psychological consequences of neurological conditions when adapted specifically for this population. Further research will help to determine when and for whom CFT may offer an optimally effective treatment approach.

Adaptations and considerations for neurological conditions including indications, contra-indications and challenges

CFT fits well within a neurorehabilitation approach in that it can be structured well according to the client's needs. CMT itself is a training approach with focus on repeated experiential practice, both within and between sessions. Smartphones can be used to record exercises during session and recordings can guide practice between sessions, until the exercises have been learned. This structured practice-based approach fits well with wider multidisciplinary neurorehabilitation input and offers a useful scaffolding of skills development for clients with cognitive difficulties. For clients with memory and executive functioning difficulties, it is important to spend time developing strategies to actively prompt clients to practice CMT exercises. Smartphone reminders and alerts can be usefully employed for this purpose. Clients can also pre-program daily texts to themselves as a prompt to bring to mind their emerging compassionate perspective (see Ashworth et al., 2011 for an example). The authors are also aware that clients may struggle to practice outside of sessions for many reasons beyond cognitive difficulties, thus an important part of the process is reflecting with clients on these experiences with the CFT *it's not your fault* perspective in order to support clients to feel de-shamed in this context and be able to find the best way forwards in bringing compassion practice to their daily lives.

CFT can be used both in both one-to-one and group therapy formats. The authors have used both formats with individuals with neurological conditions (Ashworth et al., 2015). As has been noted earlier, CFT is a relatively new approach with clients with neurological conditions so it is hard to determine what, if any length of intervention may be most effective and individual differences play a vital role in this decision making. From the authors' experiences, it differs considerably based on the individuals; however one-to-one therapy has varied from a minimum of 16 sessions up to a maximum of 40 sessions (see Ashworth et al., 2011; Ashworth, 2014; Ashworth et al., 2015 for examples applied to neurological conditions). Group interventions have varied from a two-hour session for eight weeks to 12 weeks, but without further research recommendations are difficult to ascribe.

CFT was initially developed for those with pervasive experiences of shame and self-criticism, and the evidence is emerging to support its utility with these particular groups of individuals. These experiences are frequently present in those following NC, which provides a clear rationale for use with this specific group. Given that following NC, individuals often face lifelong challenges and adjustment-related distress, learning CMT skills that can enable them to deal with these in the long run could be very beneficial. Again, longitudinal research is needed to explore this possibility. It is also possible that CMT could provide a means of developing protective skills for those who are initially lacking in awareness who may then start to develop some awareness leading to a dip in mood (see Ashworth, 2014 for a more in-depth discussion of this topic). The evidence to date (albeit it limited and sparse) suggests that CFT can be useful for individuals with neurological conditions with heightened self-criticism associated with psychological distress; however this needs confirmation with much larger scale trials.

Given the relative 'newness' of the application of CFT to those with neurological conditions, it is difficult to determine who may not benefit from such an approach in this population; however the following considerations are highlighted based on the authors' clinical experience, of which many may be universal to other therapeutic approaches. Clients with motivation issues will need to be assessed carefully as clients are required to engage with exercises within and between sessions in order to gain benefits – it may be that motivational work needs to be considered as a pre-cursor to the therapy. Additionally, given that CFT utilises practices from mindfulness, it is important to consider whom it might contra-indicated for here, e.g., caution needs to be taken with anxiety as the evidence for this is not well supported in wider populations (see chapter on mindfulness for further consideration of this point). As with any psychotherapy approach, one would also need to carefully consider the type and severity of neuropsychological difficulties of the client on their ability to engage with talking therapy. For examples of considerations of neuropsychological profiles and adaptations of CFT based on clients' profiles see Ashworth et al. (2011) and Ashworth (2014). Furthermore, it would be recommended that one seeks supervision from a clinician who is experienced in the approach when considering CFT for those individuals with long-term historical trauma and attachment issues combined with significant emotion dysregulation as a result of the neurological condition, as ensuring the client feels safe and secure and can be contained is fundamental when there is the possibility of opening up these attachment systems.

In relation to this aforementioned issue of opening up attachment systems, a key area that CFT aims to address within the therapy is fear, blocks and resistances (FBRs) to compassion (Gilbert, 2019). It us unsurprising that those high in shame and self-criticism may struggle to access compassion and experience FBRs. Research has highlighted that fears of compassion are strongly associated with depression, shame and self-criticism (Kirby, Day, & Sagar, 2019). Therefore, the CF therapist will focus on understanding and addressing these FBRs as a key part of therapy.

Clinical reflections on using CFT with people with neurological conditions

It is the authors' experiences that CFT can be a useful approach with individuals with neurological conditions. It offers a way of working towards being free from feelings of shame and self-criticism, which may be barriers to improving their wellbeing. Furthermore, given that CFT draws on the neuroscience of emotions and more broadly on the role of executive control of emotions as a key part of the psycho-education and de-shaming process, we believe that this approach can be useful in conceptualising psychological distress following ABI as well as for intervention and management of such difficulties. In particular the three circles model has been found to be a simple and engaging way to help people with neurological conditions makes sense of their emotional experiences as well as being 'light' on cognitive load (Ashworth et al., 2015).

As a third-wave approach, CFT is situated within the cognitive-behavioural therapy tradition, albeit with a primary focus on cultivating self-compassion rather than cognitive restructuring of negative thought patterns. In the authors' experience, a positive indication for CFT would be situations where clients struggle to benefit from cognitive restructuring, usually expressed as follows: 'I get it but I just don't feel it' (see Ashworth et al., 2011 for an illustrative case example). Within the Interacting Subsystems Model (Teasdale & Barnard, 1993), this is conceptualised as change at the propositional level (contents of cognition) not translating into change at the implicational level (emotional 'felt sense'). CFT offers a structured way to access the implicational level via CMT exercises and enhances the client's ability to reflect on how various ways of relating to the self (self-compassionate versus self-critical) produce immediate and observable shifts in embodied emotional experience. CFT overlaps with mindfulness-based approaches in terms of approach, method and focus on shifting the relationship to distress. However, mindfulness approaches typically require a reasonably high level of self-regulation and initiation in order to maintain the level of practice required to yield gains. This can present a barrier for clients with acquired cognitive difficulties. Within CFT, the incorporation of mindfulness-based exercises within the structured compassionate mind training component seems to scaffold the development of mindfulness skills in a helpful way for clients with neurological conditions.

Given that CFT is a focused psychotherapy, rather than a particular therapy orientation, one of the advantages is that it draws on existing therapeutic skills from other specific traditional psychotherapies. This means that therapists can draw from a wide variety of their pre-existing skills and tools in helping clients build compassion. In CFT, personal therapist practice is also very important; this we feel is an additional advantage in that the therapist embodies compassion in the room (whilst still being human and fallible!) as well as values the practice of it in their own lives. This enables greater synergy or attunement which we feel significantly affects the relational aspect of the therapy enabling us to connect and be present with the client in a way that is humanising. In addition to this, some therapists may experience self-criticism or shame in relation to working therapeutically with clients with neurological conditions (e.g., feeling 'not good enough' to support change, feeling frustrated at lack of progress or slowness of therapy). Being able to bring compassion to this can help shift blocks to therapy for the therapist, who can then feel empowered to work more effectively with the client. Personally, I (FA) have found CFT to be a profoundly powerful experience in both my personal life and professional practice. I find that I enjoy my life and work even more with the development and nurturing of my own compassion and have better tools to deal with the suffering that life brings. Using this approach with clients with neurological conditions has enabled me to have a much greater understanding of their experiences, and I have been inspired by many of these individuals in having the courage to turn towards their own suffering and pain and learning to use compassion to work with it. I think this is captured well in a quote from a client who took part in our mixed one-to-one and group CFT study (as cited in Ashworth et al., 2015, p. 14):

> Without being compassionate to myself, I would still not have had the tools to be able to stop myself going into the deep depression stages. I would have perhaps had tools to not get into the situations so much but, like I said earlier, there are times where you are still going to muck it up and it's how you respond to that, that is where the compassionate mind really comes into its own. Paul

Case example

The case example used here is from the Neurorehabilitation Activity Programme (NAP), which is designed as a holistic self-management group for people with long-term neuro-disability, based on the principles of Compassion Focused Therapy. This group was run by Dr Clara Murray, clinical psychologist (coauthor), Vicky Haworth, occupational therapist and Lynette Sue, neurological physiotherapist.

Background and rationale

The programme was developed as an interdisciplinary initiative, incorporating occupational therapy, physiotherapy and psychological interventions. The rationale for combining functional and psychological elements was explained to participants in terms of the interconnectedness of body and mind, of mental fitness and physical fitness. The development and delivery of the group was undertaken as a pilot project, with the aim of evaluating the applicability of CFT principles and techniques in a group-based programme for people living with long-term neuro-disability. The pilot group was run in a local community centre in a deliberate move away from a medical or clinic setting. The eight-week programme involved a weekly two-hour session, with exercises to be completed between sessions.

Assessment and formulation

The programme was open to people living with a long-term neurological condition (18 months +). The inclusion of all neurological conditions provided a diversity of experience, as well as highlighting overarching points of commonality in facing the challenges of neuro-disability. Five participants were assessed and included in the group with a range of neurological conditions including multiple sclerosis (two females), cerebrovascular accident (CVA) (two males) and post-surgical acquired brain injury (one female). Participants ranged in age from 50 to 59, and the time since diagnosis ranged from 18 months to 19 years.

Group aims

The group aimed to enable participants to identify meaningful functional goals, understand their condition and learn to positively influence their functioning in relation to these goals through targeted exercises and increased awareness in everyday activities. The group also aimed to support participants to renegotiate their relationship to their neuro-disability, through feedback and a compassionate reflective group process.

Functional goal-setting: focusing on what matters

Using an adapted measure (based on the Canadian Occupational Performance Measure, Law et al., 1990), participants were supported to identify areas of their lives, which they were motivated to work on improving, and up to five meaningful goals within key areas. On a 0–10 scale, participants rated both their performance and their satisfaction in relation to goals at the beginning and end of the programme.

Participants' concerns about their functional abilities to carry out tasks related to their personal goals were addressed in the goal-setting process. Mobility was an important goal for all participants and was associated with a valuing of independence. Physical balance was also highlighted as being important for moving safely and confidently when carrying out daily tasks. Participants received one-to-one physiotherapy and occupational therapy input relating to their specific functional goals. Goals included being able to use a snooker cue in the context of right-sided weakness (participant with CVA), improving transfers to reduce fatigue and maintain independence (participant with MS), improving vestibular function in order to return to riding a motorbike (participant with cerebellar CVA).

Physical fitness: mastering the seven primary movements of everyday activity

Participants were individually assessed by the physiotherapist to establish their baseline physical abilities and to identify key aspects related to their functional goals. The programme was structured around educating participants about the seven primary movements (bend, squat, lunge, twist, push, pull, walk) and fine motor control, which form the building blocks of all functional movement patterns. Each week a primary movement was introduced in the first half of the session. Exercises to enhance this movement were discussed, demonstrated and performed. A range of functional tasks involving this movement were considered and practiced. Video feedback was used to enable participants to observe and review their own performance in discussion with the physiotherapist. Participants were encouraged to increase their awareness of the primary movement as they went about daily tasks that week, as a way of enhancing their movement efficiency. A written summary was provided about each movement, its functional importance and exercises for improving it.

> A little something each week which I was able to pick up on. Not "you must do these exercises" but "how can we incorporate this into your daily living". Each time I stand up, I try to do it the proper way to exercise my thighs. It has to be making a difference.
>
> *Ion*

> I found it very positive. I've told you I'm rubbish at doing exercises and things, but the whole attitude wasn't "well that's no good at all" . . . it was "well it doesn't matter, if you're going to build it into your life a bit more then that's good". All the feedback was on the positive side rather than "you're not doing it right, you should be doing this."
>
> *Sheila*

The importance of nutrition was also covered and discussed during the mid-session break, accompanied by healthy snacks.

Mental fitness: cultivating compassion

The following elements of CFT were integrated into the group programme:

Psycho-education

Participants were introduced to core principles of Compassion Focused Therapy, including Gilbert's (2009) definition of compassion, to approach, engage, and understand suffering, along with a commitment to work towards alleviating it. Participants were introduced to Gilbert's (2009) three circles model, which describes three interconnected affect regulation systems: the threat system, the drive/achievement system and the safety/soothing system.

Finding mental balance between these systems in order to maintain psychological wellbeing was emphasised and equated with the need for physical balance in carrying out everyday activities. It was acknowledged that this balance is quite tricky to achieve in daily life, as our culture reinforces a tendency to primarily rely on the drive/achievement system to down-regulate threats. Over time, this pattern can lead to under-recruitment and underdevelopment of the soothing/safety system.

Participants were encouraged to generate examples of the different modes of mind associated with the activation of each system, based on their own experiences. Participants were able to use the three circles model (Figure 5.1) to make sense of shifts in their emotional experience in response to being confronted with the loss of functional abilities. The following quote illustrates an example of attempting to down-regulate threat system activation (e.g., 'to stop feeling like a burden') by 'doing' or 'achieving' something.

> It's very demoralising – makes me think "why am I bothering?" I'm doing all this work and getting nowhere fast . . . like a duck under water – nice and calm on the top and paddling like hell underneath . . . and going nowhere. I'd do all the housework in one day, and then I'm exhausted and thinking "why?. . . . I've got all week!"
>
> *Peter*

The difficulties encountered when striving to achieve plunges people back into the threat system, with associated feelings of failure, inadequacy and frustration. The three circles model succinctly formulates this 'boom and bust' pattern, which is so common for people who are struggling with reduced cognitive capacity and/or neurological fatigue. The model also reveals how the activation of the threat system in response to fatigue can trigger a barrage of self-criticism. This can trap people in a loop of absorbing negative affect, which is difficult to exit because of reduced executive capacity. Participants described the challenge of managing these inner emotional experiences and a sense that nobody around them was able to fully understand.

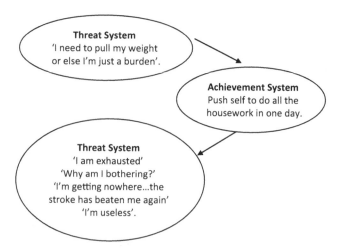

FIGURE 5.1 Example formulation using the Three Circles Model: maintenance cycle

Other people have sympathy for you but they don't know what it's like. You've been thrust from being normal into being disabled just like that. It's a shock – one minute you're in this world, the next minute you're in that world – it's hard to get used to.

Martyn

For the first time I was able to verbalise and share my anger, frustrations and disappointments with people who understood where I am coming from, this in itself was like throwing off a heavy weight.

Amanda

The three systems model (Figure 5.2) allowed these experiences to be explored in a de-shaming and normalising way. It also provided the rationale for using exercises to engage and develop the soothing system in order to down-regulate threats, reframe expectations and restore balance across the three systems.

Compassionate mind training (CMT)

The following compassionate mind training exercises were used (see Gilbert, 2010c for description):

1   Soothing rhythm breathing
2   Body scan
3   Safe place exercise

The exercises were taught and practiced in session to provide participants with the experience of doing something that helps them to feel better in the moment

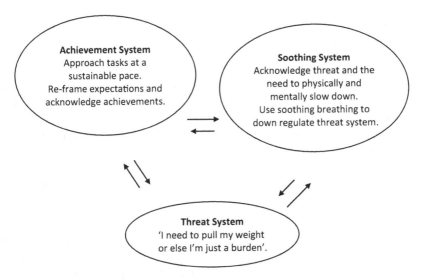

FIGURE 5.2 Example formulation using the Three Circles Model

by reducing physiological arousal associated with threat system activation. Participants used the three circles formulation to identify situations where they could use the exercises to exit frustrating patterns of boom and bust, driven by the threat system. Four out of the five participants engaged well with these exercises and subjectively reported feeling immediate benefits of relaxation and feelings of contentment. One participant noted 'Meditation. I can see the value but it's not for me'. Participants were given a CD with guided audio versions of these exercises recorded specifically for the group. They were encouraged to practice the guided exercises at home initially with the CD, progressing to self-guided practice once they were familiar with the exercise.

Compassionate action: putting compassion into action

A necessary step towards adjustment was supporting participants to confront their difficulties in a way that felt safe and comfortable for them. Video-feedback of the activities was used to enhance participants' awareness and understanding of their current level of functioning. In this way, participants were encouraged to compassionately witness their own struggle, and to open themselves to working on whatever aspects would help them to move forward.

> When I watched [other participants] walk. . . . I thought "yeah, you're doing that wrong and I actually do that". . . . I could [imagine] me doing it and thought "I've got to do this". So it was good for me to see somebody else doing what I do and I was able to see how to correct it.
>
> *Ion*

Building a compassionate sense of identity: relating to self, others and distress/disability in a more compassionate way

Throughout the programme, a reflective group process was facilitated, in which therapists also participated. Each session began with a 'check-in' where all present shared something about their past week, such as what changes they had hoped to make and how this had gone. This was intended to break down barriers around competence, expertise and disability and to model Gilbert's (2009) fundamental common humanity principle. We are all in the same boat, and our experiences (including negative emotional experiences) are an understandable part of being human, as opposed to something shameful arising from some personal flaw or shortcoming.

> It was nice the way that professionals have been prepared to give your own thoughts and experiences rather than just expecting us to do it. Participating as someone receiving rather than just delivering the programme.
>
> *Sheila*

The atmosphere is one of the most important things . . . If I feel comfortable in a situation, I pick the other things up better. If I feel vulnerable or uncomfortable, everything else closes off . . . I had been doing exercises, but the ones I've been doing since this started – they've helped.

Peter

Meeting other people with the same or similar problems who are in the same boat.

Martyn

As participants became comfortable in the group (circa week 3), their capacity to offer compassionate reflections and feedback to each other increased. Participants became adept at delivering honest, helpful feedback in a nonjudgmental or critical way. The group began to develop its own compassionate mind, which in turn supported individual participants to build a compassionate sense of identity and to be more encouraging towards themselves.

Somebody else telling you things but not being critical – that is a big thing. "Oh I noticed this or you were doing that" but not in a critical way.

Peter

Participants giving tips to each other. Asking someone who has done it "I did that but I got over it by doing this". . . . I never thought of that!

Martyn

We were honest and open about where we were mentally and physically. We encouraged one another regarding our progress; even the smallest achievements were recognised. Friendships were built, laughter shared and a chance to finally acknowledge the "New Me", a similar but modified version of the "Old Me".

Amanda

Evaluation and Outcomes

Outcome evaluation was based on:

1   Progress with functional goals, based on participants' subjective ratings of their performance and level of satisfaction pre- and post-intervention.
2   Psychological wellbeing, based on self-rating questionnaire measures (Hospital Anxiety & Depression Scale (HADS, Zigmond & Snaith, 1983); Forms of Self-Criticism and Reassurance Scale (FSCRS, Gilbert, Clarke, Hempel, Miles, & Irons, 2004; Baiao, Gilbert, McEwan, & Carvalho, 2015)
3   Subjective feedback of participants, based on a facilitated feedback session.

Data for one participant was incomplete. For three participants, mean ratings for performance and satisfaction across identified goals showed modest improvements from baseline (1 to 2 points on the 1–10 scale). Three participants described having altered their expectations of themselves in regard to task performance as a direct result of what they had learned in the group.

> And I'll try and find that balance, because it's taken [me] quite a while, but I've finally realised that the harder I work, it doesn't necessarily mean the faster I'll get better – it can be counter-productive. Because I think I've really been working too hard, I've been doing far too much. I'm starting to bring it down a little bit and it's better, cause I don't get that boom and bust – which is really bad for me.
>
> *Peter*

> It has really driven home to me how much I do need to incorporate it all into my day-to-day stuff, because my main fear with this condition is severe deterioration. So I'm just hoping that if I can do the things we've been doing here, I will at least slow that process down a bit.
>
> *Sheila*

Group analyses on questionnaire measures revealed a statistically significant reduction in levels of anxiety ($p = 0.046$), but no significant changes were noted on other questionnaire measures at a group level. Pre- and post-HADS ratings were analysed individually for clinically significant changes. A reduction in total HADS score of 1.5 has been established as the minimal important difference criterion in a comparable chronic health population (Puhan, Frey, Buchi, & Schunemann, 2008). Two participants exceeded this criterion, with pre-post reductions in total HADS score of 4 and 11 respectively, suggesting robust clinically significant changes. Both participants demonstrated reductions in anxiety (from 'severe' to 'moderate' range and from 'mild' to 'normal' range), and one participant showed a reduction in depression (from 'moderate' to 'mild' range). The two participants whose scores did not show clinically significant change had scored within the normal range at baseline.

Reliable change on the FSCRS was analysed using the procedure outlined by Evans, Margison, and Barkham (1998). Three participants showed reductions in self-criticism and increases in self-reassurance; however only one participant met the reliable change criterion in relation to increased self-reassurance (RCC = 6.99).

Qualitative feedback was elicited from participants in a facilitated discussion in the final session, and direct quotes included here were transcribed from this discussion. One participant could not attend the final session and submitted her reflections on the programme in writing.

Discussion

Pilot data from the programme suggests that the elements of compassion focused therapy included in this adjustment and self-management programme were experienced as helpful by participants. Based on participants' feedback, these elements appeared to contribute significantly to participants' felt sense of safety within the group and openness to confront challenging aspects of living with neuro-disability. Participants described reframing their expectations and evaluations of their own performance in a positive way. Objective measures showed reductions in anxiety and improvements in functional performance. Combining physical, functional and compassion-focused therapy interventions appears to be beneficial in supporting adjustment to long-term neuro-disability. In particular, this approach is recommended for people who are experiencing psychological distress associated with adjustment difficulties. Within this pilot group, participants with higher scores on the HADS appeared to engage best and benefit most from compassionate mind training techniques and exercises. Four out of five participants specifically commented on how the atmosphere and orientation of the group had been helpful to them in learning about what they can do to move forward. These preliminary findings suggest that CFT offers a relevant and useful platform for adjustment and self-management interventions in neurorehabilitation.

> First, let me say that I did not want to be part of a group that was different. I wanted to be part of a "Normal Group", however I felt I did not meet the full criteria any more, I almost fitted but couldn't express my true feelings in case I made people feel uncomfortable. I am no longer the person I used to be and need to accept the new me.
>
> Don't get me wrong, I still get angry and frustrated but I am able to use the strategies' taught in the group and contact the friends I have made. There is light at the end of the tunnel, it may not be the light you were looking for but a new and challenging one. The goals you set at the beginning of the programme change along the way. I think we all came to realise that mental wellbeing is the most important because without a healthy mental outlook, nothing is really achievable.
>
> *Amanda*

Summary and conclusion

As a third-wave therapy approach, CFT focuses on how people relate and respond to their experience rather than necessarily aiming to directly change the experience. Drawing on Buddhist philosophy, the model distinguishes between pain and suffering – between what happens to us, and how we struggle with what has happened to us. The authors have found this approach to be particularly helpful to clients who are struggling with the emotional consequences of neurological conditions and coming to terms with the reality of long-term neuro-disability. As clinicians, we often meet clients who are grappling with unwelcome shifts in roles and identity and fighting to reclaim the 'old me'. In the authors' experience, the key features of CFT that appear to work well for people with neurological conditions include the following:

- Simple, clear cross-sectional formulation which clients can relate to
- Practical exercises linked to formulation which enable clients to down-regulate threat responses, shame and self-attack and to develop more compassionate responses
- Clinicians modelling an acknowledgment of their own vulnerability and humanity
- Relating differently to the struggle – cultivating tools for facing an uncertain and difficult future without losing hope, renegotiating identity and life goals, facing the pain and grief associated with losses
- Relating differently to the self and to others – A key outcome from the Neurorehab Activity Program was participants seeing value in other people with neurological conditions, and in turn feeling genuinely valued by others, so that they could recognize their own on-going worth, alongside their disability. This is consistent with findings indicating that forming new supportive relationships outside of one's existing network is associated with post-traumatic growth following acquired brain injury (Powell, Gilson, & Collin, 2012).

In conclusion, CFT offers clients with neurological conditions a framework for confronting their circumstances and their distress with compassion and with a commitment to reduce their own suffering. As a structured psychotherapy, it provides useful tools for engaging with a different and uncertain future.

References

Ashworth, F. (2014). Soothing the injured brain with a compassionate mind: Building the case for compassion focused therapy following acquired brain injury. *Neuro-Disability and Psychotherapy, 2*(1–2), 41–79.

Ashworth, F., Clarke, A., Jones, L., Jennings, C., & Longworth, C. (2015). An exploration of compassion focused therapy following acquired brain injury. *Psychology and Psychotherapy: Theory, Research and Practice, 88*(2), 143–162.

Ashworth, F., Evans, J. J., & McLeod, H. (2017). Third wave cognitive and behavioural therapies: Compassion focused therapy, acceptance and commitment therapy and positive psychotherapy. In B. A. Wilson, J. Winegardner, C. M. van Heugten, & T. Ownsworth (Eds.), *Neuropsychological rehabilitation: The international handbook* (pp. 327–339). New York: Routledge/Taylor & Francis Group.

Ashworth, F., Gracey, F., & Gilbert, P. (2011). Compassion focused therapy after traumatic brain injury: Theoretical foundations and a case illustration. *Brain Impairment, 12*(2), 128–139.

Baiao, R., Gilbert, P., McEwan, K., & Carvalho, S. (2015). Forms of self-criticism/self-attacking and self-reassuring scale: Psychometric properties and normative data. *Psychology & Psychotherapy: Theory Research & Practice, 88*(4), 438–452.

Campbell, I. N., Gallagher, M., McLeod, H. J., O'Neill, B., & McMillan, T. M. (2019). Brief compassion focused imagery for treatment of severe head injury. *Neuropsychological Rehabilitation, 29*(6), 917–927.

Carter, C. S. (1998). Neuroendocrine perspectives on social attachment and love. *Psychoneuro Immunology, 23*, 779–818.

Craig, C., Hiskey, S., Royan, L., Poz, R., & Spector, A. (2018). Compassion focused therapy for people with dementia: A feasibility study. *International Journal of Geriatric Psychiatry, 33*(12), 1727–1735.

Depue, R. A., & Morrone-Strupinsky, J. V. (2005). A neurobehavioural model of affiliative bonding. *Behavioural and Brain Sciences, 28*, 313–395.

Evans, C., Margison, F., & Barkham, M. (1998). The contribution of reliable and clinically significant change methods to evidence-based mental health. *Evidence Based Mental Health, 1*, 70–72.

Freeman, A., Adams, M., & Ashworth, F. (2015). An exploration of the experience of self in the social world for men following traumatic brain injury. *Neuropsychological Rehabilitation, 25*(2), 189–215.

Gracey, F., & Ownsworth, T. (2012). The experience of self in the world: The personal and social contexts of identity change after brain injury. In J. Jetten, C. Haslam, & S. A. Haslam (Eds.), *The social cure: Identity, health and well-being* (pp. 273–295). Hove and New York: Psychology Press.

Gilbert, P. (2005). *Compassion: Conceptualisations, research and use in psychotherapy*. Hove, UK: Routledge.

Gilbert, P. (2009). *The compassionate mind*. London: Constable & Robinson.

Gilbert, P. (2010a). *Compassion focused therapy: Distinctive features*. London: Routledge.

Gilbert, P. (Ed.). (2010b). Compassion focused therapy [special issue]. *International Journal of Cognitive Therapy, 3*, 95–210. https://doi.org/10.1521/ijct.2010.3.2.95

Gilbert, P. (2010c). *Training our minds in with and for compassion: An introduction to concepts and compassion focused exercises*. Retrieved from http://wtm.thebreathproject.org/wp-content/uploads/2016/03/COMPASSION-HANDOUT.pdf

Gilbert, P. (2014). The origins and nature of compassion focused therapy. *British Journal of Clinical Psychology, 53*(1), 6–41.

Gilbert, P. (2019). Explorations into the nature and function of compassion. *Current Opinion in Psychology, 18*, 108–114.

Gilbert, P., & Allan, S. (1998). The role of defeat and entrapment (arrested flight) in depression: An exploration of an evolutionary view. *Psychological Medicine, 28*(3), 585–598.

Gilbert, P., Clarke, M., Hempel, S., Miles, J. N., & Irons, C. (2004). Criticizing and reassuring oneself: An exploration of forms, styles and reasons in female students. *British Journal of Clinical Psychology, 43*, 31–50.

Gilbert, P., & Miles, J. N. (2000). Sensitivity to social put-down: It's relationship to perceptions of social rank, shame, social anxiety, depression, anger and self-other blame. *Personality and Individual Differences, 29*(4), 757–774.

Hagger, B. F. (2011). *An exploration of self-disclosure after traumatic brain injury*. Unpublished manuscript. Birmingham, UK: Department of Psychology, University of Birmingham.

Haslam, C., Holme, A., Haslam, S. A., Iyer, A., Jetten, J., & Williams, W. H. (2008). Maintaining group memberships: Social identity continuity predicts well-being after stroke. *Neuropsychological Rehabilitation, 18*(5–6), 671–691.

Jones, L., & Morris, R. (2013). Experiences of adult stroke survivors and their parent carers: A qualitative study. *Clinical Rehabilitation, 27*(3), 272–280.

Kirby, J. N. (2017). Compassion interventions: The programmes, the evidence, and implications for research and practice. *Psychology and Psychotherapy: Theory, Research and Practice, 90*(3), 432–455.

Kirby, J. N., Day, J., & Sagar, V. (2019). The "Flow" of compassion: A meta-analysis of the fears of compassion scales and psychological functioning. *Clinical Psychology Review, 70*, 26–39.

Kirsch, P., Esslinger, C., Chen, Q., Mier, D., Lis, S., Siddhanti, S., & Meyer-Lindenberg, A. (2005). Oxytocin modulates neural circuitry for social cognition and fear in humans. *The Journal of Neuroscience, 25*, 11489–11493.

Law, M., Baptiste, S., McColl, M., Opzoomer, A., Polatajko, H., & Pollock, N. (1990). The Canadian occupational performance measure: An outcome measure for occupational therapy. *Canadian Journal of Occupational Therapy, 57*(2), 82–87.

Leaviss, J., & Uttley, L. (2015). Psychotherapeutic benefits of compassion-focused therapy: An early systematic review. *Psychological Medicine, 45*(5), 927–945.

LeDoux, J. (1998). *The emotional brain*. London: Weidenfeld & Nicolson.

MacBeth, A., & Gumley, A. (2012). Exploring compassion: A meta-analysis of the association between self-compassion and psychopathology. *Clinical Psychology Review, 32*(6), 545–552.

MacDonald, K., & MacDonald, T. M. (2010). The peptide that binds: A systematic review of oxytocin and its prosocial effects in humans. *Harvard Review of Psychiatry, 18*, 1–21.

Neff, K. D., & Beretvas, S. N. (2013). The role of self-compassion in romantic relationships. *Self and Identity, 12*(1), 78–98.

O'Neill, M., & McMillan, T. M. (2012). Can deficits in empathy after head injury be improved by compassionate imagery? *Neuropsychological Rehabilitation, 22*(6), 836–851.

Powell, T., Gilson, R., & Collin, C. (2012). TBI 13 years on: Factors associated with post-traumatic growth, *Disability & Rehabilitation, 34*, 1461–1467.

Poz, R. (2014). Facing degeneration with compassion on your side: Using compassion focused therapy with people with a diagnosis of a dementia. *Neuro-Disability and Psychotherapy, 2*(1–2), 80–99.

Puhan, M. A., Frey, M., Buchi, S., & Schunemann, H. J. (2008). The minimal important difference of the hospital anxiety and depression scale in patients with chronic obstructive pulmonary disease. *Health & Quality of Life Outcomes, 6*, 46.

Riley, G. A., Brennan, A. J., & Powell, T. (2004). Threat appraisal and avoidance after traumatic brain injury: Why and how often are activities avoided? *Brain Injury, 18*(9), 871–888.

Shields, C., & Ownsworth, T. (2013). An integration of third wave cognitive behavioural interventions following stroke: A case study. *Neuro-Disability and Psychotherapy, 1*(1), 39–69.

Teasdale, J., & Barnard, P. (1993). *Affect, cognition and change*. Hove, UK: Lawrence Erlbaum Associates.

Yarnell, L. M., & Neff, K. D. (2013). Self-compassion, interpersonal conflict resolutions, and well-being. *Self and Identity, 12*(2), 146–159.

Zigmond, A. S., & Snaith, R. P. (1983). The hospital anxiety and depression scale. *Acta Psychiatrica Scandinavica, 67*(6), 361–370.

6

POSITIVE PSYCHOTHERAPY FOR NEUROLOGICAL CONDITIONS

Jonathan J. Evans and Breda Cullen

In this chapter we will argue that a psychotherapy approach based on principles derived from the field of positive psychology may be useful in the treatment of mood disorder symptoms and distress in people with neurological conditions, including acquired brain injury. This therapy approach has been termed 'positive psychotherapy' (PPT; Seligman, Rashid, & Parks, 2006).[1]

From the outset we note that at the present time there is insufficient evidence to confirm whether or not PPT is effective in treating mood disorder symptoms and distress after brain injury. This is because there are insufficient evaluations of the efficacy/effectiveness of PPT from which to draw firm conclusions. We will, however, outline why we believe PPT has the potential to be useful and look at the evidence for the effectiveness of PPT interventions in other populations, as well as the evidence to date that does relate to people with neurological conditions.

Positive psychology

Positive psychology (PP) is concerned with wellbeing – what it is, how to measure it and how to increase it (Seligman, 2011, p. 12). The term 'happiness' is often associated with PP. Indeed, the book that set out to define the field of positive psychology was titled, *Authentic Happiness* (Seligman, 2002). More recently, however, Seligman has noted that he dislikes the term happiness because 'it underexplains what we choose' and 'the modern ear immediately hears "happy" to mean buoyant mood, merriment, good cheer and smiling' (Seligman, 2011, p. 10). Seligman's point is that the construct of wellbeing is much broader than the concept of happiness, at least when happiness is defined narrowly in terms of having a cheerful mood.

Theories of positive affect and wellbeing are not new. Philosophers have for centuries considered questions of what constitutes happiness, wellbeing and a satisfied life. Well before positive psychology emerged as a distinct field of study in the late 1990s, psychologists had argued that it is as important to understand what constitutes positive mental health as it is to understand negative mental health states, or psychopathology. This historical context was acknowledged by PP pioneers such as Peterson and Seligman (2004), who discussed the influence of the work of theorists such as Marie Jahoda (1958), who had argued that six processes contribute to positive mental health: acceptance of oneself, growth/ development/ becoming, integration of personality, autonomy, accurate perception of reality and environmental mastery. However, it is clear that the huge increase in attention to theory and assessment of wellbeing, and interventions to increase wellbeing, has been driven by the early work of Seligman in his colleagues in the late 1990s and early 2000s.

The thrust of Seligman's argument for a focus on wellbeing was that, in relation to the treatment of psychological disorders such as depression, research and clinical practice has developed interventions (both pharmacological and psychological) that have at best rather modest effects on symptom relief, with benefits that typically fade over time (Seligman, 2011, p. 48). The outcome measures for trials of interventions to treat depression focus, quite reasonably, on reduction of symptoms of depression. But this means that a successful treatment is defined only in terms of feeling less depressed. There was a relative lack of focus on increasing wellbeing (other than an implicit assumption that reducing mental ill health is improving wellbeing). Seligman, however, argued that perhaps an explicit focus on improving wellbeing could lead to changes in psychological health that would not just reduce the symptoms of depression but lead to sustainable changes in behaviour, thinking and feeling that would reduce the likelihood of a return to depression. Seligman was not just interested in finding new ways to treat people who were depressed but also interested in whether the wellbeing of the average person could be increased. Assuming that wellbeing is not just the absence of depression, is it possible to move people from 'average wellbeing' to much greater wellbeing? So that was the starting point for positive psychology. But before thinking about how to improve wellbeing, the task was to understand more about what actually constitutes 'wellbeing'. This led Seligman and colleagues to develop a model that aimed to define the core psychological characteristics that plausibly capture the experience of wellbeing. The initial version of this model (Duckworth, Steen, & Seligman, 2005) had three elements, referred to as 'forms of living': the pleasant life, the engaged life and the meaningful life. In 2011, Seligman extended this to five components in the PERMA model.

Defining wellbeing

PERMA refers to Positive emotion, Engagement, Relationships, Meaning and Achievement. Positive emotion includes the experience of pleasure, feelings of comfort, warmth, etc. Engagement relates to being actively engaged in activities that challenge, but do not overwhelm, using personal *character strengths*, or traits to meet those challenges. The concept of engagement is influenced by Csikszentmihályi's (1990) idea of 'flow', defined as the experience of being completely involved in an activity for its own sake, involving a challenging activity that requires skills, with clear goals and feedback, focused attention and a sense of control, which is sometimes associated with the experience of loss of the sense of the passage of time. Flow is also discussed by Yeates (this volume) in relation to Tai Chi mind-body interventions for neuro conditions. The inclusion of positive relationships in the PERMA model highlights the fundamental importance of social relationships to wellbeing; positive relationships are authentic connections through which we feel loved, supported and valued by others. Meaning was defined as belonging to, and serving, positive institutions, which are things that are considered to be 'bigger than the self' (Seligman, 2011, p. 17) including families and communities, volunteering, public service and so on. The final component is accomplishment, which refers to the pursuit of success for its own sake, reflecting the desire to achieve.

Evans (2011) suggested that Seligman's model of wellbeing may be useful in thinking about the impact of brain injury on mental health, as part of a psychological formulation process. Brain injury may disrupt the ability to experience pleasure (including sensory pleasure when smell or taste are impaired, experiencing sexual pleasure, deriving enjoyment from previously enjoyed activities or experiencing a sense of optimism or contentment). It may not be possible to engage in activities (leisure, vocational) that provided opportunities to experience flow. Relationships are very frequently disrupted. Activities that previously gave a sense of meaning and purpose may no longer be accessible. Finally, it may be difficult, or impossible, to achieve goals that a person was pursuing prior to their brain injury. Thus, for many people, acquired brain injury, and indeed other neurological conditions, could be seen to limit access to key aspects of life that previously gave a sense of wellbeing. In this context it is unsurprising that the rate of depression is elevated in people who have experienced brain injury (Jorge et al., 2004), stroke (Hackett & Pickles, 2014) and other neurological conditions.

Nevertheless, we also know that depression is not inevitable. Indeed, some people experience post-traumatic growth (PTG) after brain injury (Collicutt McGrath & Linley, 2006; Rogan, Fortune, & Prentice, 2013). A systematic review by Grace, Kinsella, Muldoon, and Fortune (2015) summarised the findings of eight quantitative studies of PTG following acquired brain injury, most of which had used the Post Traumatic Growth Inventory (PTGI). There was evidence that brain injury survivors experienced growth on the five factors of the PTGI, namely appreciation of life, relating to others, personal strength, new possibilities and spiritual change. These findings were echoed in a more recent study of brain injury survivors by Karagiorgou and Cullen (2016). Amongst people who have not experienced a brain injury or the onset of a neurological condition, there is perhaps a risk of making an assumption that wellbeing will inevitably be worse for those who have and remain worse in perpetuity. Clinicians and families may, however, benefit from understanding more about those who cope well in the context of adversity in order to understand how to better help those who struggle.

Another important concept in PP is that of character strengths. Character strengths are considered to be positive human traits that transcend cultures (Peterson & Seligman, 2004). A set of 24 character strengths has been defined that are considered to fall into six broader categories: Wisdom (e.g., curiosity, creativity), Courage (e.g., bravery, honesty), Humanity (e.g., love, kindness), Temperance (e.g., forgiveness, humility), Justice (e.g., leadership, teamwork) and Transcendence (e.g., gratitude, hope). Rashid and Seligman (2018) have speculated that perhaps psychological disorders could be conceptualised in terms of either a lack or excess of one or more of these character strengths. This idea builds on the earlier argument of Peterson (2006) that both underuse and overuse of character strengths might indicate negative functioning and psychopathology, whereas 'optimal' use reflects positive functioning. There is limited empirical research in this area; one study, by Freidlin, Littman-Ovadia, and Niemiec (2017), found that both overuse and underuse of social intelligence were associated with social anxiety. In addition, overuse of humility and underuse of zest, humour and self-regulation were also associated with social anxiety.

Much more research is clearly needed to determine whether conceptualising psychological disorders in relation to over- or underuse of character strengths is helpful. In relation to brain injury and other neurological conditions it might be argued that the common cognitive and physical consequences may limit the ability to use, or express, character strengths in the same way as before the injury or onset of the condition. People who are able to maintain the opportunity to express their strengths may be protected from distress, whilst those who are unable to express their most valued strengths may be vulnerable to distress. Haslam et al. (2008) studied people recovering from stroke and found that life satisfaction was related to maintenance of social group membership. They noted that 'cognitive failures compromised well-being in part because they made it hard for individuals to maintain group memberships post stroke' (p. 671). Loss of a sense of belonging could be considered in PERMA terms, as a loss of relationships and meaning but also in terms of loss of the opportunity to express character strengths such as love, kindness, social intelligence, teamwork and humour, amongst others. Character strengths vary between people, which means that the same deficits and functional consequences of a brain injury may have very different impact on different people, depending on how those deficits and disabilities affect the expression of each person's unique character strengths.

We argue that a core task for neuropsychological rehabilitation is to enable people with neurological conditions to maximise their psychological health, and to achieve this it is helpful to think not only in terms of reducing depression, anxiety or distress but also to focus very explicitly on improving wellbeing. This is the aim of positive psychotherapy.

Positive psychotherapy

As noted, the first task for the positive psychologists was to understand what constitutes and influences the experience of wellbeing. A second task was to be able to measure wellbeing and the various domains of wellbeing reflected in the theoretical models. The third task was to address the question of whether wellbeing can be improved using interventions derived from PP theory.

Over the years, a number of PP measurement tools have been developed and, to varying degrees, evaluated in terms of their reliability and validity. These include questionnaires that examine aspects of positive emotion, engagement, meaning and overall life satisfaction, as well as character strengths inventories. Very few of these tools have been validated in people with brain injury, though in our recent pilot trial of Positive Psychotherapy (Cullen et al., 2018) we evaluated the Authentic Happiness Inventory (AHI) and the Brief Strengths Test (both developed by Christopher Peterson and available at www.authentichappiness.sas. upenn.edu) with brain injury survivors. There remains a need for further validation of measures of wellbeing for people with neurological conditions.

Efforts to develop PP interventions began by examining whether the wellbeing of people who were not suffering from mental health conditions could be improved. Seligman, Steen, Park, and Peterson (2005) developed exercises designed to improve wellbeing, which they tested in a randomised controlled trial (RCT) with 577 adult participants. Participants completed one of five exercises or a placebo task. They found that most tasks, including the placebo, led to increased happiness immediately post-intervention, but two interventions showed improvements that persisted at three and six months. These were the 'three good things' and 'using signature strengths in a new way' interventions. In the 'three good things' exercise, participants were asked to write down three things that went well each day for one week. Additionally, they were asked to provide an explanation for why each good thing happened (with the aim of highlighting how the good thing came about). The intervention referred to as 'using signature strengths in a new way' involved participants completing an inventory of character strengths and receiving individualised feedback about their top five ('signature') strengths. They were then asked to use one of these top strengths in a new and different way every day for one week. These specific exercises have been incorporated, along with others, into an intervention package referred to as Positive Psychotherapy (PPT; Seligman, Rashid, & Parks, 2006; Rashid & Seligman, 2013; Rashid & Seligman, 2018). Other exercises include a focus on gratitude, forgiveness, satisficing versus maximising (accepting 'good enough' rather than constant striving for better), savouring, positive communication in relationships (active constructive responding), hope, optimism and posttraumatic growth and altruism. In its most recent form (Rashid & Seligman, 2018), PPT is a 15-session intervention, with each session introducing a core PP concept, accompanied by tasks and 'homework' activities designed to enable participants to implement the key strategies in their everyday lives.

PPT has been used in a variety of contexts, and has been delivered in one-to-one, group and online delivery formats. It has been used with nonclinical populations, as well as with people who are depressed, or have other physical or psychological conditions. Two meta-analyses of studies that included positive psychology interventions have been published in the last decade. Sin and Lyubomirsky (2009) reported a meta-analysis of 25 studies that examined the impact of positive psychology interventions on people with depression and found a medium mean effect size (r = .31). They noted that the interventions were most effective with self-selecting participants and increased in effectiveness with older age of participants. Individual therapy was superior to group interventions and self-administered interventions. Longer interventions (e.g., > 8 weeks) were better than shorter (e.g., ≤ 4 weeks) interventions. Bolier et al. (2013) reported a review of 39 randomised studies that included PPT interventions and found overall modest effects of interventions on measures of depression and wellbeing (standardised mean difference 0.20–0.34). They also highlighted that many of the studies were low in methodological quality. Furthermore, only a small number were aimed at participants with clinical levels of psychological difficulties (e.g., depressive symptoms).

PPT has also been adapted for use with people living with a diagnosis of psychosis (Slade, Brownell, Rashid, & Schrank, 2017). In the same way that Evans (2011) argued that PPT could be relevant for people after brain injury, Slade et al. have argued that an explicit focus on wellbeing may inform the development of new approaches to supporting the recovery of people who have experienced psychosis. The concept of recovery has been prominent in psychiatric rehabilitation over the last two decades, and Slade et al. suggest that there is a lot of overlap between conceptualisations of recovery and wellbeing, noting the definition of recovery from Anthony (1993) that refers to 'a deeply personal, unique process of changing one's attitudes, values, feelings, skills and/or roles. It is a way of living a satisfying, hopeful and contributing life even within the limitations caused by illness' (p. 14). Prior to developing their PPT intervention for psychosis recovery, Slade et al. developed a framework of wellbeing based on a systematic review of how wellbeing has been measured in this clinical population and on an empirical study of how people with a history of psychosis experience wellbeing and how it might be enhanced. In addition they investigated potential challenges to applying PPT interventions with people who have experienced psychosis, and how such challenges might be met with modifications to the PPT programme. As a result Slade et al. developed an 11-session group-based PPT programme (later revised to 13 sessions), with 90-minute sessions, including five minutes at the beginning and end to listen to music and a ten-minute mid-session refreshment break. Many of the original PPT intervention elements were included, though some were considered too challenging and were removed (e.g., satisficing versus maximising; altruism).

PPT for psychosis recovery was evaluated in a pilot randomised controlled trial (WELLFOCUS PPT; Schrank et al., 2016). Schrank et al. randomised

94 participants to either the 11-session PPT intervention or a treatment as usual (TAU) control condition. TAU included assessment and interventions that were standard in the multidisciplinary teams from which participants were recruited. Mean attendance rate was 54.2% of sessions and 55% of the intervention group completed the intervention. Drop-out rate did not differ between conditions. The primary outcome measure was the Warwick-Edinburgh Mental Wellbeing Scale (WEMWBS). A wide range of other measures of wellbeing were also administered. Schrank et al. reported that on baseline-follow-up change measures the PPT group showed statistically significant improvement on the WEMWBS and a number of the other wellbeing measures, whereas the control group showed no changes on any of the measures. However, an intention-to-treat analysis found no significant effect of intervention group on the WEMWBS at follow up after adjusting for baseline scores, though there were significant effects on three other measures (a measure of wellbeing, a psychiatric symptom scale and a measure of depression). In addition the views of participants were obtained via interview or focus group (Brownell, Schrank, Jakaite, Larkin, & Slade, 2014). Brownell et al. reported that feedback about the PPT group was positive throughout. Components reported to be helpful by a majority of participants included the savouring, three good things and personal strengths exercises. Other elements that were also reported as helpful, but noted to be challenging, included the forgiveness and gratitude exercises, with a small number of participants not being able to complete them because of triggering difficult emotions. Overall, Schrank et al. (2016) concluded that the WELLFOCUS trial had provided initial evidence for the feasibility and acceptability of the intervention, but further work was needed to optimise effectiveness. The clinicians' manual (Slade et al., 2017) incorporates revisions of this PPT intervention for psychosis recovery, which needs to be evaluated in a larger scale RCT.

Positive psychotherapy in brain injury and other neurological disorders

Evans (2011) had argued that the PP idea of 'building what's strong rather than fixing what's wrong' is consistent with person-centred, goal focused neuropsychological rehabilitation that emphasises the importance of enabling people to increase participation in valued activities (Hart & Evans, 2006). It was also suggested that there may be potential for application of some of the specific interventions developed within the PP/PPT context within brain injury rehabilitation settings.

Andrewes, Walker, and O'Neill (2014) investigated the use of PPT interventions in an inpatient brain injury rehabilitation hospital, using a group format. Their study involved ten patients with severe, very severe or extremely severe brain injury who were randomly allocated to a PPT intervention or a TAU control group. The PPT group ran for 12 weeks and provided a general introduction to mindfulness, gratitude, values and strengths. Within this, the two main interventions were the three good things journal and 'signature strengths' exercises. Andrewes et al. reported that on a measure of happiness (the Authentic Happiness Inventory) participants in the PPT group were happier compared to baseline and the control group immediately following the two-week 'three good things' intervention, though this was not statistically significant at the end of the 12-week intervention. Following the signature strengths exercise, there was no significant change on the outcome measure being used (the Head Injury Semantic Differential Scale) although Andrewes et al. suggested that PPT participants tended to report a more positive self-concept after the intervention. Given the very small sample size it is necessary to be cautious about the results. Nevertheless, it was reported that participants appeared to find the group format and sessions acceptable and, with an appropriate level of individualised support, it was feasible to use these interventions in a group format with patients who had suffered severe brain injuries.

We (Cullen et al., 2018) developed an eight-session, one-to-one PPT intervention for outpatients with brain injury which was evaluated in a pilot randomised controlled trial (the PoPsTAR trial). Participants in the control arm received usual care that could include any psychological intervention routinely offered by the clinical service. Participants in the PPT arm received usual care plus the PPT intervention. We selected and adapted a number of elements from Rashid and Seligman's PPT programme that we felt would be most appropriate to people with brain injury and also included psychoeducation about brain injury. The session topics included:

- Session 1: Information about stroke/brain injury and introduction to Positive Psychology
- Session 2: Character strengths (learning about character strengths and about under- and overuse, identifying five 'signature' strengths, and learning to use them in new ways)
- Session 3: Gratitude, Savouring and Three Good Things (a focus on identifying things for which a person is grateful, expressing gratitude, savouring positive experiences and introduction to the three good things journal)
- Session 4: Mid-point summary and review
- Session 5: Optimism, hope and personal growth (completing a 'one door closes, another opens' exercise; understanding personal growth after brain injury)
- Session 6: The gift of time (altruism and a focus on taking the time to help another person or a cause you feel strongly about)
- Session 7: The full life (a focus on engagement and flow and setting goals to facilitate opportunities for engagement/flow)
- Session 8: Final summary and plan for future maintenance

In the PoPsTAR trial, the primary outcome measures related to evaluating the feasibility of a trial of PPT in this population: recruitment rate, treatment adherence and retention at 20 weeks from baseline. Secondary outcomes included the test-retest reliability of the Authentic Happiness Inventory (AHI) and the Signature Strengths inventory, change in Depression Anxiety Stress Scales (DASS-21) scores at 20 weeks from baseline, changes in AHI, Mayo Portland Adaptability Index 4 (MPAI-4) and the Modified Caregiver Strain Index scores at 20 weeks from baseline and ratings of participants' and therapist's experience of treatment delivery.

A total of 27 participants were randomised, with 14 assigned to Positive Psychotherapy, of whom eight completed treatment. On the whole, reasons for noncompletion were not related to the intervention. One participant did report finding it distressing talking about difficulties and did not wish to continue, though this may have occurred with any talking therapy. Overall retention in the study was 63%, which is comparable with studies of other psychological therapies. The intervention was rated as feasible to deliver with excellent fidelity and was acceptable to participants. Completion rates for homework tasks were high: across all participants who attended at least one session that involved homework, 74% of tasks were fully or partly completed. All eight participants who attended the full treatment programme completed at least 70% of their assigned homework. Being a feasibility study, this trial's primary purpose was not to examine outcomes with regard to changes in levels of distress or wellbeing. Effect size estimates in terms of standardised mean difference between intervention and control groups as assessed by change scores on the DASS anxiety ($d = 1.09$), DASS depression ($d = 0.73$), DASS stress ($d = 1.10$) and AHI ($d = 1.11$) were in the directions anticipated, but the small scale of this study means that these should not be interpreted as indicators of efficacy. Given the results from PoPsTAR, Cullen et al. concluded that a full scale RCT of brief positive psychotherapy for emotional distress following brain injury was justified and feasible.

In a related study, Karagiorgou, Evans, and Cullen (2018) investigated posttraumatic growth (PTG) experiences of people who had participated in the PoPsTAR trial. Four people who had undergone the PPT intervention and three people in the control arm were interviewed individually using a semi-structured interview focused on five factors of PTG. Participants were asked questions regarding their lives before and after the brain injury, how the brain injury occurred and how it changed their lives, focusing on positive changes. They were then asked to review a PTG questionnaire that they had completed at the end of the trial and explain their interpretation of the statements that they had endorsed strongly or not endorsed. What emerged from thematic analysis were six themes relating to PTG shared by participants from both the PPT and control arms. These related to personal strength (resilience and adapting to change), appreciation of life, relating to others (increased closeness to others), optimism and a positive attitude, feeling fortunate compared to others (things could have been worse) and positive emotional/behavioural changes (feeling calmer). In addition, two themes were expressed only by PPT participants: lifestyle improvements (actively changing lifestyle) and new possibilities (the opportunity to do new things). One theme was expressed only by a participant in the control arm, which related to increased spirituality. It was noted that participants also mentioned negative aspects of life since their injury as well as positive growth-related changes. This is not surprising of course, and it is worth emphasising that PPT does not suggest ignoring or denying negative aspects of life post-injury but rather focusing more attention to experiences that give a sense of wellbeing and learning to act in a way that promotes wellbeing.

Resilience training and brain injury

Resilience is an important concept in relation to recovery from any trauma and has been a key focus of the work of positive psychologists. Resilience refers to recovering quickly from difficulties, which implies recovering back to a pre-difficulty (pre-trauma) state. Like the concept of post-traumatic growth discussed earlier, resilience is sometimes used to describe how a person may be able not only to resist, or recover from, the (common) negative consequences of trauma but also to experience a renewed appreciation of being alive, greater personal strength, improved relationships, changes in life priorities and so on. This raises the question of whether it is possible to facilitate resilience post-trauma and also whether it is possible to train people to have greater resilience so that they will be able to recover from trauma should they experience it in future.

Seligman (2011) described a 'Master Resilience Training' programme, which has been rolled out to US Army soldiers. The programme – Comprehensive Soldier Fitness (CSF) Training – involves learning to manage thinking (using some standard cognitive-behavioural therapy techniques), dealing with catastrophic thoughts, 'hunting the good stuff' (i.e., using the three good things journal), using character strengths to overcome challenges, building strong relationships via active constructive responding style, effective praise and assertive communication. The programme was not evaluated using standard clinical trial methodology, and this has prompted some criticisms. Seligman (2011) noted that his original plan was to evaluate the programme in an initial pilot trial but the army Chief of Staff, convinced by related PP based study evidence, decided simply to roll it out. An evaluation of the programme was published (Lester, Harms, Herian, Krasikova, & Beal, 2011) that compared outcomes for a group of 6739 soldiers who received the training with 3218 who did not. The report concluded that there were statistically significant differences on the main outcome measure of resilience (the Global Assessment Tool) that favoured the training group, leading to an overall conclusion that 'There is now sound scientific evidence that Comprehensive Soldier Fitness improves the resilience and psychological health of Soldiers' (p. 1). However, the report has been heavily criticised. In a working paper, Eidleson and Soldz (2012) argued that the study of Lester et al. did not measure relevant outcomes, was methodologically flawed in terms of not controlling effectively for various potential confounders and in terms of the approach to data analysis and also did not acknowledge potential risks associated with CSF training. The jury is perhaps still out on whether CSF training can prevent psychological distress in soldiers.

Kreutzer et al. (2018) developed and evaluated an intervention to improve resilience after brain injury, with resilience being defined as positive adaptation in the face of a traumatic event. The intervention, which Kreutzer at al. characterise as 'borrowing from the field of positive psychology' with a focus on skill building and positive attributes rather than personal limitations and impairments, involved seven one-hour one-to-one sessions conducted over a five-week period covering topics such as emotional regulation, stress management, problem solving and communication. The intervention was evaluated in an RCT with 160 participants allocated to either the intervention (n = 83) or a wait-list control (n = 77), with follow up analysis being conducted on n = 75 (intervention) and n = 73 (control) participants. The primary outcome measure was a self-report measure of resilience (the Connor-Davidson Resilience Scale; CD-RISC), with secondary measures of psychological distress (Brief Symptom Inventory-18; BSI-18), stress (13-item stress test) and adaptability (MPAI-4). Kreutzer et al. found a statistically significant and clinically meaningful improvement on the measures of resilience (CD-RISC) and emotional distress (BSI-18) for the resilience group compared to the wait-list group. For other measures there were statistically significant differences between the groups, but the level of change did not meet a priori criteria for clinically meaningful changes. The major limitation for this study was use of a wait-list design which severely limits conclusions that can be drawn in relation whether the specific resilience interventions were responsible for any changes over time. However, there was clearly sufficient indication that further evaluation of the programme would be appropriate.

Other positive psychology interventions

A variety of other interventions characterised as 'positive psychological interventions' have been used with people with a wide range of neurological disorders. Lim, Low, and Tang (2018) reported a systematic review of positive psychological interventions (PPIs) for neurological disorders. Their definition of PPIs was relatively broad, being activities or therapies that aim to enhance the positive, for instance positive feelings, cognition, and/or behaviours, with an explicit focus on wellbeing. Lim et al. suggested that savouring, mindfulness, gratitude and optimism were considered exemplary strategies in relation to wellbeing. Their systematic search identified 31 studies (21 controlled studies) relating to ten different neurological conditions. Most interventions were group based. The vast majority of these studies (n = 24) included mindfulness-based techniques, with much smaller numbers of other types of intervention. Lim et al. made a very strong recommendation for mindfulness but in addition made strong recommendations in relation to positive savouring, use of life summaries and hope interventions. However, given the acknowledged methodological limitations in many of the studies it seems we should be very cautious about drawing conclusions for any intervention other than mindfulness, which has a much stronger evidence base.

Conclusions

There is a strong rationale for drawing upon the theoretical framework of positive psychology and the specific techniques of positive psychotherapy in the treatment of mood disorder symptoms and distress in people with neurological conditions. At the present time there is insufficient evidence to draw firm conclusions about the efficacy of PPT for people with brain injury, stroke or other neurological conditions. Meta-analyses of PPT studies with people with depression and other forms of psychological distress (but without a neurological condition) indicate that PPT can be effective at reducing symptoms, with modest effect sizes. For those with brain injury, or psychosis, recent feasibility trials have had positive results, finding that PPT interventions are feasible to deliver and acceptable to patients. Larger scale trials are now needed.

Note

1 For clarity it should be noted that this form of positive psychotherapy is not the same as Peseschkian's positive psychotherapy (see Dobiała and Winkler (2016) for a discussion of similarities and differences).

References

Andrewes, H. E., Walker, V., & O'Neill, B. (2014). Exploring the use of positive psychology interventions in brain injury survivors with challenging behaviour. *Brain Injury, 28*(7), 965–971.

Anthony, W. A. (1993). Recovery from mental illness: The guiding vision of the mental health system in the 1990's. *Psychosocial Rehabilitation Journal, 16*, 11–23.

Bolier, L., Haverman, M., Westerhof, G. J., Riper, H., Smit, F., & Bohlmeijer, E. (2013). Positive psychology interventions: A meta-analysis of randomized controlled studies. *BMC Public Health, 13*, 119.

Brownell, T., Schrank, B., Jakaite, Z., Larkin, C., & Slade, M. (2014). Mental health service user experience of positive psychotherapy. *Journal of Clinical Psychology, 71*, 85–92.

Collicutt McGrath, J., & Linley, P. A. (2006). Post-traumatic growth in acquired brain injury: A preliminary small scale study. *Brain Injury, 20*(7), 767–773.

Csikszentmihalyi, M. (1990). *Flow.* New York: Harper & Row.

Cullen, B., Pownall, J., Cummings, J., Baylan, S., Broomfield, N., Haig, C. . . . Evans, J. (2018). Positive PsychoTherapy in ABI rehab (PoPsTAR): A pilot randomised controlled trial. *Neuropsychological Rehabilitation, 28*(1), 17–33.

Dobiała, E., & Winkler, P. (2016). "Positive psychotherapy" according to Seligman and "positive psychotherapy" according to Peseschkian: A comparison. *International Journal of Psychotherapy, 20*(3), 5–17.

Duckworth, A. L., Steen, T. A., & Seligman, M. E. P. (2005). Positive psychology in clinical practice. *Annual Review of Clinical Psychology, 1*, 629–651.

Eidleson, R., & Soldz, S. (2012). Does comprehensive soldier fitness training work? CSF fails the test. *Coalition for an Ethical Psychology*, Working Paper No. 1.

Evans, J. J. (2011). Positive psychology and brain injury rehabilitation. *Brain Impairment*, *12*(2), 117–127.

Freidlin, P., Littman-Ovadia, H., & Niemiec, R. M. (2017). Positive psychopathology: Social anxiety via character strengths underuse and overuse. *Personality and Individual Differences*, *108*, 50–54. https://doi.org/10.1016/j.paid.2016.12.003

Grace, J. J., Kinsella, E. L., Muldoon, O. T., & Fortune, D. G. (2015). Post-traumatic growth following acquired brain injury: A systematic review and meta-analysis. *Frontiers in Psychology*, *6*, 1162.

Hackett, M. L., & Pickles, K. (2014). Part I: Frequency of depression after stroke: An updated systematic review and meta-analysis of observational studies. *International Journal of Stroke*, *9*(8), 1017–1025. https://doi.org/10.1111/ijs.12357

Hart, T., & Evans, J. J. (2006). Self-regulation and goal theories in brain injury rehabilitation. *Journal of Head Trauma Rehabilitation*, *21*(2), 142–155.

Haslam, C., Holme, A., Haslam, S. A., Iyer, A., Jetten, J., & Williams, W. H. (2008). Maintaining group memberships: Social identity continuity predicts well-being after stroke. *Neuropsychological Rehabilitation*, *18*, 671–691.

Jahoda, M. (1958). *Current concepts of positive mental health*. New York: Basic Books.

Jorge, R. E., Robinson, R. G., Moser, D., Tateno, A., Crespo-Facorro, B., & Arndt, S. (2004). Major depression following traumatic brain injury. *Archives of General Psychiatry*, *61*(1), 42–50. https://doi.org/10.1001/archpsyc.61.1.42

Karagiorgou, O., & Cullen, B. (2016). A comparison of post-traumatic growth after acquired brain injury or myocardial infarction. *Journal of Loss and Trauma*, *21*, 589–600.

Karagiorgou, O., Evans, J. J., & Cullen, B. (2018). Post-traumatic growth in adult survivors of brain injury: A qualitative study of participants completing a pilot trial of brief positive psychotherapy. *Disability and Rehabilitation*, *40*(6), 655–659. https://doi.org/10.1080/09638288.2016.1274337. PMID:28068845

Kreutzer, J. S., Marwitz, J. H., Sima, A. P., Mills, A., Hsu, N. H., & Lukow, H. R. 2nd. (2018). Efficacy of the resilience and adjustment intervention after traumatic brain injury: A randomized controlled trial. *Brain Injury*, *32*(8), 963–971.

Lester, P. B., Harms, P. D., Herian, M. N., Krasikova, D. V., & Beal, S. J. (2011). *The comprehensive soldier fitness program evaluation. Report #3: Longitudinal analysis of the impact of master resilience training on self-reported resilience and psychological health data.* Publications of Affiliated Faculty: Nebraska Public Policy Center, 32. Retrieved from http://digitalcommons.unl.edu/publicpolicyfacpub/32

Lim, K.-S., Low, W.-Y., & Tang, V. (2018). Positive psychological interventions for neurological disorders: A systematic review. *The Clinical Neuropsychologist*, *33*(3), 490–518. https://doi.org/10.1080/13854046.2018.1489562

Peterson, C. (2006). The values in action (VIA) classification of strengths. In M. Csikszentmihalyi & I. S. Csikszentmihalyi (Eds.), *A life worth living: Contributions to positive psychology* (pp. 29–48). New York: Oxford University Press.

Peterson, C., & Seligman, M. E. P. (2004). *Character strengths and virtues: A classification and handbook*. Washington, DC: American Psychological Association.

Rashid, T., & Seligman, M. E. P. (2013). Positive psychotherapy. In R. J. Corsini & D. Wedding (Eds.), *Current psychotherapies* (10th ed., pp. 461–498). Belmont, CA: Cengage.

Rashid, T., & Seligman, M. E. P. (2018). *Positive psychotherapy: Clinician's manual*. Oxford: Oxford University Press.

Rogan, C., Fortune, D. G., & Prentice, G. (2013). Post-traumatic growth, illness perceptions and coping in people with acquired brain injury. *Neuropsychological Rehabilitation*, *23*(5), 639–657. https://doi.org/10.1080/09602011.2013.799076

Schrank, B., Brownell, T., Jakaite, Z., Larkin, C., Pesola, F., Riches, S. . . . Slade, M. (2016). Evaluation of a positive psychotherapy group intervention for people with psychosis: Pilot randomised controlled trial. *Epidemiology and Psychiatric Sciences, 25*, 235–246.

Seligman, M. E. P. (2002). *Authentic happiness.* New York: Atria.

Seligman, M. E. P. (2011). *Flourish: A new understanding of happiness and wellbeing and how to achieve them.* London: Nicholas Brealey Publishing.

Seligman, M. E. P., Rashid, T., & Parks, A. C. (2006). Positive psychotherapy. *American Psychologist, 61*, 774–788.

Seligman, M. E. P., Steen, T. A., Park, N., & Peterson, C. (2005). Positive psychology progress: Empirical validation of interventions. *American Psychologist, 60*(5), 410–421.

Sin, N. L., & Lyubomirsky, S. (2009). Enhancing wellbeing and alleviating depressive symptoms with positive psychology interventions: A practice friendly meta-analysis *Journal of Clinical Psychology: In Session, 65*, 467–487.

Slade, M., Brownell, T., Rashid, T., & Schrank, B. (2017). *Positive psychotherapy for psychosis: A clinician's guide and manual.* London: Routledge.

Yeates, G. N. (in press). Mind-body interventions for neurological conditions. In G. N. Yeates & F. Ashworth (Eds.), *Psychological therapies in neuropsychological rehabilitation.* Hove, UK: Psychology Press.

7

ATTACHMENT-BASED PSYCHOTHERAPIES FOR PEOPLE WITH ACQUIRED BRAIN INJURY

Giles N. Yeates and Christian E. Salas

Introduction

This chapter explores the contribution of attachment theory in both (1) the conceptualisation of negative emotional and social outcomes following adult acquired brain injury, and also (2) guiding therapeutic responses for both individual survivors (psychodynamic psychotherapy) and couples/family interventions (emotionally focused therapy, EFT). Following a theoretical introduction to attachment process and their neurobiological substrate, this literature is used to identify both pre- and post-injury factors that contribute to emotional and social disconnection between survivors and their significant others. Finally, a model of cumulative socioemotional dysregulation and disconnection is presented to summarise these applied concepts.

Attachment: a universal theory for mammals with or without brain injury

Attachment has been defined as an inborn system (Bowlby, 1969; Panksepp, 1998) that organizes physiological and brain regulation (Schore, 2003; Fonagy et al., 1995), improving the chances of infant survival by motivating them to seek proximity to parents (Bowlby, 1973), this, as a mean to reestablish safety and reduce states of tension (Fonagy et al., 1995). From a developing point of view, attachment facilitates the establishment of interpersonal relationships, which are the social context where the immature brain of the child uses the mature functions of the parent's brain to organize and scaffold its own processes (Hofer, 1994). It is important to clarify that attachment has a central role not only during childhood but also influences and orchestrates behaviour during adulthood. According to Siegel (1999), in children the search for physical proximity allows protection from situations that are a source of danger (hunger, attacks from predators, separation) and modulates disorganising mental states. In adults, particularly during moments of stress, the activation of this system is frequently observed in relation to the search of availability of specific attachment figures (parents, partners), as a source of comfort, advice and support.

A central finding of attachment theory is that, based on repeated interaction with attachment figures, children develop expectations in relation to the nature of these interactions (Fonagy et al., 1995). These expectations are later transformed into mental representations or 'working models' (Bowlby, 1979). Working models function as schemas or blueprint for expected *interpersonal* patterns of behaviour and communication (Ainsworth, 1993). In other words, these schemas facilitate information processing and influence decision making by quickly predicting possible outcomes based on previous experience. Another relevant aspect in attachment theory is that the history of interactions with carers and the way they respond to individual's needs will have a key role shaping personality, emotional regulation and self-regulation (Calkins & Leerkes, 2004; Cassidy, 1994; Feeney, 2006). This refers to the *intrapersonal* dimension of attachment, which will influence the self-to-self interaction during stressful or threatening situations.

Research on infant and adult attachment has offered substantial evidence to support this idea and has extensively described different attachment patterns, its behavioural and physiological correlates as well as its representational transformation throughout adolescence and adulthood (Ainsworth, Blehar, Waters, & Wall, 1978; Crittenden & Landini, 2011; George, Kaplan, & Main, 1985; Main, 1995; Main & Solomon, 1990). Attachment theory's focus on emotional experience, embodiment and physicality of loving relationships has stimulated a range of policy changes in hospital care, education, family support and adoption services, amongst others (Crittenden, 1995). Panksepp (1998) has substantiated and validated Bowlby's initial observations of innate attachment behaviours in several mammalian species and has identified a shared mid-brain neuro-anatomical substrate (involving the periaqueductal grey, nucleus accumbens, hypothalamus and anterior cingulate cortex) shared by mammals that functions to elicit attachment distress behaviours in infants and corresponding pro-nurturing responses from care-givers. A complimentary framework by Porges (2009) has identified the key role of the ventral polyvagal complex in the socially affiliative behaviour (e.g., eye gaze, posture, vocal gestures and mouth movements) of a mammal to elicit pronurturing responses from caregivers and affiliative responses from peers.

This work highlights the profound dimension of attachment experience, emotions, motivations and interpersonal behaviours for all mammals, including humans. So both the neuroscientific study of brain-behaviour relationships following neuropathology and the development of clinical interventions and services based on this knowledge would be fundamentally incomplete should an attachment perspective not be formally included. Unfortunately, in the field of neuropsychological rehabilitation this is the case, since literature using an attachment perspective to understand the diagnosis, case formulation and treatment of people with *acquired* brain injury is still scarce (Bowen, Yeates, & Palmer, 2010; Yeates, 2013; Salas, 2012). This situation contrasts markedly with the development of theoretical and technical models in the rehabilitation of people with *progressive* neurological disorders (e.g., Browne & Shlosberg, 2006; Cheston, Thorne, Whitby, & Peak, 2007; Miesen, 1992; Kokkonen, Cheston, Dallos, & Smart, 2014; Nelis, Clare, & Whitaker, 2014). The main goal of this chapter is to address such theoretical and technical gap, highlighting how the inclusion of attachment theory could impact on clinical neuropsychological perspectives on brain injury and neurorehabilitation.

Attachment as a dimension of post-injury adjustment and adaptation

Adult ABI has been traditionally researched using individualistic frames of reference (Bowen et al., 2010). However, the widespread strain and breakdown of significant relationships of all kinds post-injury, with accompanying emotional distress for all concerned (Perlesz, Kinsella, & Crowe, 2000; Yeates, 2009), signposts the primacy of the emotional and relational in brain injury outcomes, and therefore the potential relevance and usefulness of Attachment Theory. Nevertheless, it is striking that no research paper of this kind exists in the brain injury literature.

It is not controversial to formulate many events in life post-injury as attachment crises. For the survivor, a subjective sense of disorientation and loss of control in life is common, with simultaneous experiences of psychological distress such as anxiety, depression, anger and traumatic stress (Coetzer, 2009). The injury forces sudden vulnerability on survivors as abilities are lost or undermined, and there is a new dependence on close ones who often are required to facilitate information processing, decision making or externally regulate negative emotional states (Freed, 2002; Salas, 2012; Salas et al., 2014). This core scenario post-injury has the potential to trigger positive attachment cycles of closeness and connection between survivors and their loved ones. However, this potential is commonly undermined by a range of pre-injury and injury-related factors, often influencing the escalation of distress and disconnection in survivor and significant other. These factors will be explored in turn in the following sections.

Pre-injury attachment histories of survivors and significant others

This new situation of functional limitations, and dependence from others, will be inevitably signified by the attachment history of each survivor, both interpersonally and intra-personally. Interpersonally, individuals that experienced their carers in childhood as available and sensitive to their needs will probably acknowledge after the injury the necessity of relying on others to function properly and trust them more easily. On the contrary, individuals that had problematic attachments with their carers during childhood will tend to avoid relying on people, seek support or directly reject any kind of help. Intra-personally, attachment history will shape the way that the survivor regulates negative emotions triggered by functional limitations, or the way that he/she relates to new physical or cognitive aspects of the self that emerge as a consequence of the injury. The relationship between functional/emotional adjustment post-injury and attachment history might seem obvious to the reader, but it is still a matter of debate in the field of neuropsychological rehabilitation due to a certain distrust to the psychoanalytic provenience of these ideas (for a review on such debate *see* Salas, 2014). It is important to mention here that, with the recent incorporation of Compassion Focused Therapy (Gilbert, 2005) as a psychological intervention for ABI survivors, attachment theory has gained a space in the neuropsychological rehabilitation field (Ashworth, 2014; Ashworth, Clarke, Jones, Jennings, & Longworth, 2015; Ashworth, Gracey, & Gilbert, 2011).

Considering the importance of attachment after brain injury compels us to keep in mind not only the survivor's attachment history but also the relative's. It has been described that relatives can experience 'attachment anxieties' (Freed, 2002), or emotional reactions (e.g., withdrawal/aggression), as a response to the survivors' impairments in social cognition. The survivor, as a person who may have once provided a role as a caregiver, close confident or lover ('someone who knew me better than anyone else', 'someone who used to make everything feel better') may be unable to perform the same function post-injury. In other words, a common bidirectional process by which people mutually coordinate and regulate feelings, cognitions and interactions, a process known as *extrinsic* emotion regulation (Niven, Totterdell, & Holman, 2009; Zaki & Williams, 2013), or emotion co-regulation (Butler & Randall, 2013), might be altered by the injury. This attachment dimension is critical for both emotional communication between the couple, and also their physical, sexual relationship. Both pre-injury attachment histories of survivor and partner, and the impact of post-injury changes in cognition and interpersonal behaviour can influence sexual disconnection between the couple, and their engagement with post-injury psychosexual interventions (Yeates, in press).

Injury-related challenges to attachment bonds and regulatory interpersonal patterns

Given the aforementioned presence of a shared mammalian neuro-anatomical substrate that underlies the embodied and relational experience of attachment need (Panksepp, 1998), elicitation of caring response from others and the motivated responding of the care-giver to others' attachment distress, it follows that damage to this substrate will alter and compromise attachment patterns. In ABI survivors, such damage has been associated with a range of social cognition impairments, such as problems in mentalising/theory of mind (Channon & Crawford, 2000), sarcasm detection (Channon, Pellijeff, & Rule, 2005) and other forms of social inference

(McDonald, Flanagan, Rollins, & Kinch, 2003), emotion recognition (Hornak et al., 2003), social judgment, social decision making and problem solving (Blair & Cipolotti, 2000) and interoceptive-based decision making (Bechara, Damasio, Damasio, & Anderson, 1994). Such difficulties have been empirically linked to strained relationships with significant others, including romantic partners (Blonder et al., 2012), work colleagues (Yeates et al., 2016) and even clinicians themselves (Schönberger, Yeates, & Hobbs, in press). Yeates (2013) has offered a conceptual scheme of how different social cognition impairments can differentially lead to different patterns of disconnection between survivors and romantic partners, reproduced with permission in Table 7.1.

The subjective experiences of survivor and significant other locked into these disconnection patterns are characterised by recognisable forms of attachment distress. Several authors have collected narratives portraying such disconnection patterns, as: being 'married without a husband' (Mauss-Clum & Ryan, 1981); 'the relationship and intimacy now . . . feels wrong' (Gosling & Oddy, 1999); 'the emotional side feels badly damaged. I really miss the intimacy and closeness' (Oddy, 2001). The phenomena of post-injury personality changes in survivors are experienced by observing relatives in states of attachment distress, with the psychological organisation and identities of both survivors and relatives compromised and fundamentally altered (Yeates, Gracey, & McGrath, 2008). Such fundamental changes in relational identity and psychological connection can be most confusing and distressing in the absence of change in the survivor's physical appearance or voice. Appearing, and sounding the same to others, those closest to the survivor nonetheless can experience something unfamiliar and alien and/ or a loss of continuity with the vital essence of the person they once knew. This simultaneous superficial similarity, overlapped with a disruption to familiarity/ psychological continuity, has been described as disturbing, maddening and an isolated experience for close relatives (Boss & Couden, 2002; Feigelson, 1993; Landau & Hissett, 2008; Yeates, 2008). Others, who know the survivor less well, may not be sensitive to such interpersonal alteration. These experiences, defined by insecurity, affective dysregulation and distress, are triggered and maintained by the presence of the survivor as a confusing, ambiguous attachment figure and unable to offer a regulatory interpersonal function, thereby creating confusing and ambivalent attachment experience for close relatives (Feigelson, 1993).

As a contrast to these core neuropsychological challenges to attachment patterns, other conditions have been discussed at either ends of the lifespan where, despite profound cognitive deficits/limitations, there is a preserved capacity to reach out to others for comfort and pleasure as well as remember the centrality of such interactions. Solms (2014), for example, has drawn attention to children who are born with little or no cerebral cortex. During their short lives they clearly demonstrate joy from loving interactions with others. In the case of advanced stages of Alzheimer's Disease, the communications and behaviour of patients during moments of profound disorientation and confusion have been considered

TABLE 7.1 Neuropsychological impairments following ABI and misattunement within couples' relationships (reproduced from Yeates, 2013)

Neuropsychological impairment	Form of misattunement in the couple relationship
Executive Functioning	– Differing, contradictory or unstable goals, intentions and plans, little coordination in problem solving – Difficulties anticipating problems or outcomes, generalising across scenarios to avoid future conflict – Inflexibility in responding to problems whilst maintaining a partnership focus – Problems accessing or generating abstract concepts to conceptualise the relationship – Difficulties synthesising differing aspects of contextual information to ascertain social meaning in the moment
Attention	– No joint focus of attention – No shared priority of attentional focus – No sustained focus on a social stimuli to aid comprehension
Memory	– Reduced sharing of collective memories that signify closeness and unity in the relationship between partners or in the interactions between the couple and others – Difficulties holding on to and synthesising disparate, complex socioemotional information in working memory; misunderstanding or confusion result
Language (Aphasia)	– Reduced sharing of conversation that signifies closeness and unity in the relationship, between partners or in the interactions between the couple and others – Overt barrier to communication of intentions and understanding to each other – Expression of emotional connection through words limited (but other direct embodied forms of affect expression and comprehension possibly intact)
Mentalising	– Misattunement of intentions within couple communication – Inaccurate inference of motives behind gestures and creation of confusion and conflict – Missed early opportunities for the identification of meanings in complex, paradoxical social communication, resulting in conflict escalation – Confusion of self and other perspective, conflict escalation and/or failed reconciliation – Fewer switches from intense negative affective states/communication to a meta-perspective with the relationship and/or other's experience in mind – conflict escalation
Emotion Recognition and Autonomic Responsivity	– Missed or inaccurate resonance of core affective states, conflict initiation or escalation and/or emotional distancing as a result – Delayed responses to critical emotional communication – Failed resonance in autonomic responsivity within couple communication, lack of complementary or synchronous exchanges following emotional signalling; conflict escalation or emotional distancing as a result
Social Decision Making and Behaviour	– Failure of, or ineffective application of, socially relevant knowledge to manage any given exchange within the couple or respond to conflict – Affect dysregulation and conflict initiation/escalation, failed reconciliation – Invasion of personal space and creation of tension and conflict – Ineffective use of gut-feeling during decision making for ambiguous dilemmas or choices within social communication; maladaptive influence of individual short-term gains rather than longer-term benefits for the couple relationship – Sexual dysfunction, misattunement and consequences for broader psychological intimacy between partners

from an attachment perspective by a Dutch clinical research team. Miesen (1992, 1993, 1999; Miesen & Jones, 1997) has been interested in behaviours that are often considered meaningless, inappropriate and out of place in adults, such as patients wandering, trying to get home to see their parents who have passed away decades before. These authors argue that whilst dislocated from time and place (reflective of the cortical pathology), these behaviours are profoundly meaningful for they express the activation of intact neuro-attachment systems to regulate the distress characteristic of cognitive confusion and disorientation. This regulation reflects a primitive urge to seek proximity of a person's historical caregiver, even if cognitive abilities to test the reality of the factual presence of such a figure are not effective.

Progressive social isolation as attachment dysregulation

Difficulties in preserving old, and developing new, reciprocal and nurturing attachment relationships after brain damage cannot only compromise functional and emotional adjustment but also contribute to social isolation. Social isolation is one of the most profound life changes for persons with brain damage (Sander & Struchen, 2011) and has usually been understood as the direct consequence of a decrease in work and leisure related activities. A common complaint from survivors is the loss of relationships after the injury, often feeling disappointed, frustrated and even contemptuous of close friends and loved ones dropping away from their lives post-injury (Salas, Casassus, Rowlands, Pimm, & Flanagan, 2018). Couples and families can also experience progressive social isolation as wider family and friends drop away. Both survivors and their immediate partners (and children) can end up socially isolated without others to share the emotional burden or offer ongoing support (Bowen et al., 2010; Perlesz et al., 2000). As such the shared (and at times escalating) distress of the isolated survivor and relatives post-injury is unable to be regulated and contained in the absence of others offering wider support. We believe that an attachment perspective could also enrich our understanding of this commonly observed problem.

Formulating post-ABI multifactorial cycles of attachment distress and dysregulation

All of these facets of social relationship and their disruption post-injury have been suggested by some to define the essential nature of the human condition, the primary manifestation of a brain injury in human life and the key drivers for the scope of brain injury services (Bowen et al., 2010; Coetzer, Yeates, Balchin, & Schmidt, 2018). When the aforementioned pre-injury attachment vulnerabilities, post-injury social cognition and attachment behaviour changes, responses of significant others and progressive social isolation are conceptualised as simultaneous interacting factors, a striking picture emerges of escalating cycles of distress and disconnection that both stimulate and are influenced by wider levels of relationship. This conceptualisation is presented in diagram form in Figure 7.1:

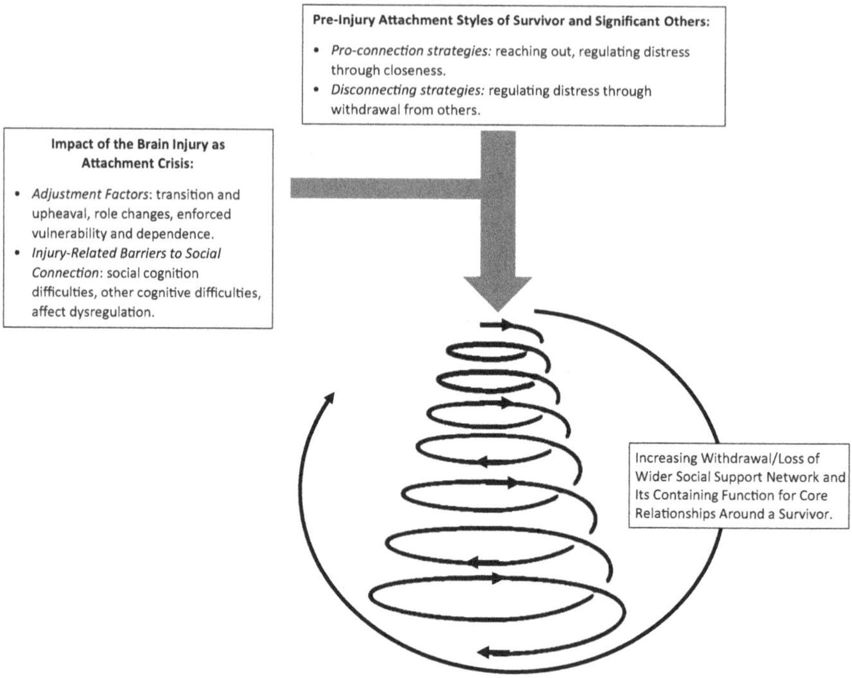

Pre-Injury Attachment Styles of Survivor and Significant Others:

- *Pro-connection strategies:* reaching out, regulating distress through closeness.
- *Disconnecting strategies:* regulating distress through withdrawal from others.

Impact of the Brain Injury as Attachment Crisis:

- *Adjustment Factors:* transition and upheaval, role changes, enforced vulnerability and dependence.
- *Injury-Related Barriers to Social Connection:* social cognition difficulties, other cognitive difficulties, affect dysregulation.

Increasing Withdrawal/Loss of Wider Social Support Network and Its Containing Function for Core Relationships Around a Survivor.

FIGURE 7.1 Cycles of attachment distress and dysregulation following acquired brain injury

If we consider a damaged neuro-anatomical substrate of attachment co-occurring alongside the social elicitation of attachment distress created by brain injury as an event impacting on a couple, family or wider social system, an ever-expanding problem emerges. That is, at moments when those distressed and vulnerable within a caregiving system need the activation of the neuro-attachment systems of all concerned, the pathology and dysfunction of those systems will overdetermine a failure of such systems to elicit the required responses and the associated attachment needs will not be met. In addition, pre-injury attachment vulnerabilities in both survivor and significant others will also overdetermine these outcomes (Yeates, in press; Yeates, Edwards, Murray, Creamer, & Mahadevan, 2013, for an example). A brain injury survivor may not be able to communicate his or her attachment needs in an adaptive way and so these may not be recognised or responded to by significant others. In turn, the attachment distress of relatives, triggered by survivor interpersonal problems, may meet with a survivor who is unresponsive and/or mistimed in their responses. Needs are unmet and distress increases over time, with this growing distress less likely to receive a proportionate nurturing response as time develops. This will occur within a wider context of diminishing social support and progressive isolation, resulting in the absence of a container to buffer and regulate the expanding, escalating distress and disconnection patterns for survivors and significant others. Such escalating distress is also likely to influence the wider social isolation, as extended family and friends may withdraw from such a bleak picture.

Attachment-influenced psychotherapies in brain injury services

Given the all-encompassing nature of these attachment dysregulation patterns and associated emotional distress, there is a central need for a core clinical response influenced and guided by attachment theory. A broad rehabilitation response influenced by attachment theory would prioritise interpersonally a caregiving relationships that *connect* survivors and significant others, and intra-personally, a focus on the relationship between the old self and new brain injured self. Good interpersonal practice examples from the existing literature include occupational therapy interventions for activities of daily living that are focused on 'family meanings' and role renegotiation (Maitz & Sachs, 1995), suggestions for physiotherapists to recruit child relatives to simultaneously optimise physical function and nurture the parent-child relationship (Daisley & Webster, 2008) and speech and language therapy work that builds on the concept of functional communication in the context of relationships for stroke survivors with aphasia (Stiell & Gailey, 2011). General guidelines on supporting relationships after brain injury have recently been published (Ahmad & Yeates, 2017). Some authors have argued that a focus solely on supporting the identity of the survivor can only proceed via enhancing their social relationships with others (Coetzer et al., 2018; Haslam et al., 2008). An example of good intrapersonal practice is Compassionate Focused Therapy (Gilbert, 2005; see also chapter 5 in this book) and the guidelines developed to facilitate positive self-to-self regulatory interactions (Ashworth, 2014; Ashworth et al., 2015; Ashworth et al., 2011).

Within this new direction for brain injury services as a whole, psychotherapy has acquired a key role: to facilitate individual and family adjustment from a *relational* point of view. This new emphasis has led clinicians to reconsider old theoretical formulations that had as a main tenet the relevance of attachment history, as well as to explore newly developed psychotherapy intervention that explicitly draw on attachment theory in both formulation of survivor difficulties and specific therapy techniques. These attachment-informed therapies prioritise both emotion and relationships, including the intrapersonal 'old me-new me' relationship and the relationship between survivor therapists and rehabilitation team, and bring these dimensions to bear on all material that a survivor shares about their lives and difficulties post-injury. Intervention techniques employed in these models are characterised by an intense focus on explicit and implicit relating and emotional patterns within the therapy room and closely following the timing of the therapeutic dialogue. In this section we will present two examples of individual and couples therapy interventions informed by attachment theory.

Individual psychodynamic therapies

It is no surprise that attachment ideas have permeated the field of neuropsychological rehabilitation through the use of psychoanalytic therapies with brain-injured patients. From its beginning, psychoanalysis proposed that personality and motivation were shaped by early relationships with carers, relationships that had a fundamental and persistent influence in present life. Psychoanalysis also noted that some of these early experiences could be 'transferred' from a significant figure of the past to people in the present (e.g., partner), and more importantly, to the therapist. Even though this idea has been considered by critics for many years as simply speculative, recent neuroscientific evidence on the 'predictive brain hypothesis' has offered substantial support. This hypothesis suggests that the brain is never at rest and its activity is never random, but constantly generating predictions based on past experience in order to interact and adjust to an everchanging environment (Bar, 2009; Pincus, Freeman, & Modell, 2007). In other words, it appears that the adult human brain does not passively perceive perceptual or social information but actively selects what to attend – based on what is relevant at the moment – and constructs meaning – constraint by what is known. Simply put: 'we don't perceive, we remember'! If we take this hypothesis to the consulting room, the old psychoanalytic idea of transference seems not so speculative after all. Human beings perceive and relate to others based on past relational and affective experiences that have been often encoded implicitly – the Attachment history. As a consequence, a patient could treat his/her therapist or expect to be treated by him/her as if relating to a significant figure from childhood, this obviously without being aware that such process was taking place. This process, due to its implicit nature, is rarely compromised by cortical damage and can be commonly observed unfolding during rehabilitation (Salas, 2012).

Historically, it was George Prigatano who put forward the idea that Attachment history had a key role in rehabilitation after brain injury. This may seem obvious now, but it was a provocative idea 20 years ago when a cognitive view of the mind and a strong emphasis on cognitive remediation prevailed in neuropsychological rehabilitation. Prigatano proposed that in order to succeed rehabilitating individuals with brain injury we should include in our case formulations their subjective experience, since it strongly influenced the rehabilitation process and how patients engaged with it (Prigatano, 1991, 1999). He called this area of intervention the 'third level of rehabilitation', separating it from therapeutic efforts aimed at restoring (first level) or compensating (second level) impaired functions (Prigatano, 2008, 2011). To him, the patient's subjective experience was composed by thoughts and feelings, which emerged in the context of their personal and socioemotional development. They reflected *attitudes towards people* that were first forged by experiences with their *primary caregivers* (mother and father). We could extend Prigatano's idea by suggesting that this third level of rehabilitation also includes *attitudes toward oneself*, which are also shaped by early relational history.

A consequence of this theoretical approach is that, when formulating a case, psychological interventions must pay attention to how the experience of acquiring a brain injury, and the many changes and losses associated to it, is signified from the particular relational history of each patient. A danger in neglecting this perspective is to devoid the patient's behaviour from any subjectivity and historicity. Thus, a patient that presents with violent anger outburst during inpatient rehabilitation can be simply understood as presenting a behavioural problem, due to disinhibition, inadequate social skills and paranoid ideation. However, when his behaviour is explored using a psychoanalytic eye it is possible to observe that he is not simply angry but, most importantly, he is offended. A valued aspect of his old self – to be respected – an aspect that was shaped by his relational history, was threatened by a social interaction in the rehabilitation ward. To understand this underlying and somewhat hidden motivation of the patient's behaviour can allow therapists to develop interventions that can engage patients in what is truly relevant for them as well as generate a sense of being understood (Prigatano & Salas, 2017).

Case Example: Mr F was a 50-year-old man who acquired a traumatic brain injury (TBI) whilst competing in a cycling race. He was a high ranked finance manager, married and father of three teenagers. As a consequence of his TBI he presented with a decreased mobility in the lower and upper left limbs, mild cognitive impairment in executive (flexibility, inhibition, monitoring) and memory functions (free recall), as well as a lack of awareness regarding his cognitive deficits. At the initial interview, seven months post TBI, he commented that he was not sure whether his accident damaged his brain or not. According to him, he came to neuropsychological rehabilitation simply because he was following orders from his physiatrist. When discussing results from the initial assessment he was adamant that his mind had never worked well before the accident, so probably that was the more likely explanation.

Even though Mr F rationalised the changes generated by his TBI, he presented intense emotional reactions to the present situation, but they were rather displaced to other events or people. He was irritable and snappy, particularly in relation to situations where he considered not to be respected as a father, or when things were not done according to his liking. He was described, by his family, as afraid when outside and constantly worried about the safety of his kids. During therapy sessions none of this came up, and he presented himself as someone cooperative and rather untroubled. The only topic that triggered emotional reactions during sessions at this initial phase of treatment was the death of his mother. She passed away two months before the accident, so due to his retrograde amnesia he had forgotten about it and was shocked by the news when he regained consciousness. Besides this, Mr F only showed signs of anxiety in relation to the outcome of our therapy sessions, since he believed that the opinion of the therapist (CS) would determine whether the physiatrist would authorise his return to work or not.

It is not our intention here to present the whole case but simply illustrate how a psychoanalytic perspective that focuses on attachment history and relational patterns can help formulating a case and develop interventions that are suited to each patient. In the case of Mr F following several sessions exploring his past history, as well as his actual experience of the changes associated to the injury, a relational pattern begun to emerge. The first piece came out when discussing his accident and feelings of insecurity. He commented:

> 'This accident was a blow, I don't even know how it happened. I had everything under control, I prepared everything as usual and I don't remember even how I fell. I know that I fell but now I realise that I was not able to do a thing. The week before I did a course on advance cycling . . . and this happens to me now, the leader of the team, the one that everyone admires.'

It appeared that the accident challenged a very basic emotional assumption in Mr F's life regarding 'having control', an aspect of his old-self that articulated relations with others and himself (we played around with the image of *grabbing a pan by the handle*, a common Chilean metaphor that refers to having control over a situation). When presenting this hypothesis to him he replied: 'I was a super man. I was the best cyclist, the leader of the team. Everyone admired me at work and asked for advice. I had never had an accident before in my life. I have always been a healthy and sporty lad'. A new element that emerged here in Mr F's narrative was the idea of feeling *invincible* and *all knowing*, aspects of the self that he considered valued and admired by others (and probably valued and admired by himself as well). At this point the therapist pointed that perhaps he now felt vulnerable and fragile, and that maybe that was the reason why he was afraid of going out or why he was worried about his kids' safety, since there was no super dad to protect them anymore. He replied: 'Sometimes I think that this must be hard for my kids – he commented- since there is no super dad anymore. Maybe they are angry at me because of that, because I was not able to avoid this accident'.

This session opened the possibility of discussing with Mr F how his accident not only changed his body and mind but also challenged his past sense of self. He agreed to the idea that part of the psychological work would imply to figure out how to live in the world without being invincible, or a superman, and how to manage the insecurity associated with the experience of vulnerability. But, what where the relational and historical roots of this emotional and hidden belief?

A couple of months into treatment Mr F came to session with his daughter and two sons. This episode offered valuable information to answer the previous question. Mr F was particularly interested in receiving help managing his 16-year-old son (Paul), who became rebellious and disrespectful after the injury. During session it was possible to observe how Mr F and Paul interacted. Paul was silent most of the session and did not speak until asked. When he begun to talk he was immediately flooded by tears and anger, evoking on the therapist an experience of disappointment and resentment. Paul talked angrily about how he felt not accepted by Mr F, how everything he did was wrong to his father eyes: his clothing, friends, what he liked. Mr F was somehow surprised by his son's reaction and made a great effort in behaving empathically to Paul's demands. He tried to put some sense onto his son by making him understand that he wanted what was *best for him*. As expected, Paul rejected his father effort by saying: 'what you think is best for me is not what I want'. After this session Mr F's relationship with his son and parenting style was explored in more detail. It was found that before the accident Paul rarely spoke or contested Mr F's instructions and orders, and that Mr F's main concern was that, without his guidance, Paul would be lost or make the wrong decisions in life. In consequence, Mr F was always on top of him, checking every homework, asking to be informed before and after every move. When asked to reflect on how he connected his way of being a dad with his experience as a son Mr F smiled:

> My dad was very strict. He always had the last word and *knew it all*. He never listened to me. It is not as if I was stupid and had no thinking of my own, or no common sense, but it was impossible to get that across. Basically I had to stay shut until I became older and left the house. Now that I think about it I see that perhaps my relationship with Paul is quite like the one I had with my dad. Honestly I wouldn't like that for him.

This session offered a key element to understand the psychological loss generated by the injury. A working hypothesis that emerged here was that Mr F's conflictive relationship with his father markedly shaped an aspect of his personality and relationship patterns with others. Somehow, Mr F became similar to his father in that he was the one who always held the answers and knew what others should do (children, cycling teammates, office colleagues). This position (the team leader/the superman/the saviour) generated a sense of control, invincibility and superiority over others that was crucial in sustaining Mr F's self-esteem. More importantly, these aspects of himself were the ones he was grieving for after the injury. And new aspects of the self, which were brought by the injury (being vulnerable, needing others, not knowing), were fiercely rejected and projected to others.

We would like to make a last comment on this case, in order to illustrate how relational patterns not only emerge during rehabilitation but most importantly are displaced (or transferred) to therapists. The relationship pattern between Mr F and the therapist unfolded quickly since the first sessions, but it was only evident months into the treatment. He commented during the initial interview: 'I come to get the opinion from an expert . . . you need to tell me if I am wright or wrong'. This was a peculiar way of describing an initial consultation, which the therapist experienced as being placed in the position of a judge. Later during the process, other interactions revealed more congruent information. The therapist noticed that Mr F used to regularly say the following phrase when discussing a topic, such as how to deal with Paul, or how to address cognitive problems: 'Please doctor you are the expert. You tell me what to do and I will do it'. During one session, he even made the following statement whilst summarising his case to a couple of students that were joining the session:

> So I did my outpatient rehab at the XX clinic. There I met my physiatrist, Dr Z, who recommended me to come and see Dr Salas. Dr Z told me that Dr Salas was the best of the best. And I only work with the best. So here I am. I have plenty confidence that with Dr Salas help I will not return to my 100% but to my 120%.

The interactions described earlier progressively showed the therapist that a relational pattern was being enacted in the therapeutic space. A pattern where one member of the dyad (the therapist) became the team leader and saviour, whilst the other (Mr F) turned into a passive and obedient patient. Interestingly, this pattern mirrored the one observed in Mr F's relationship with his son and past relationship with his father, as well as the current relationship between grandiose and vulnerable aspects of himself. In therapy, though, Mr F returned to the place of a silent and passive son, one who blindly obeyed his father. It is possible to hypothesise here that this movement helped him to tolerate the loss of his position of a superman or saviour by placing these characteristics into someone else whom will occupy that role. As the reader can imagine, to be idealised as a therapist is a risky business, since therapists are humans and humans are destined to make mistakes and fail. Idealisation is a double-edged sword, since it can quickly turn into devaluation when the person is not 'up to the standards'. It is extremely important then to address during rehabilitation these intrapersonal and interpersonal patterns before a negative therapeutic reaction is triggered. The main intervention in this case consisted in helping Mr F to become aware of this interactional pattern, particularly in relation to how he expected other people to occupy this position of 'all knowing' guide. Using metaphors from the managerial world, a world that was close to him, the possibility of considering other types of leadership was discussed. For example, horizontal forms of leadership, which were based on mutual collaboration. These metaphors resounded strongly in him, particularly as a way of understanding and modifying the relationship with his son Paul.

Emotion-focused couples therapy

Emotionally focused couples therapy (EFT) has been initially developed for couples in the general population who are experiencing distress and relationship conflict (Johnson, 2004), as part of a wave of attachment-orientated couple psychotherapies (Clulow, 2001). There is strong evidence for its efficacy for this group and where one partner has a mental health problem (Johnson, 2002). In the case of brain injury, anecdotal case reports have been described for both stroke survivors with aphasia (Stiell, Naaman, & Lee, 2007; Stiell & Gailey, 2011) and traumatic brain injury (Chawla & Kafescioglu, 2012). Yeates and colleagues

(2013) have presented a single case series quantitative evaluation of EFT for survivors of acquired brain injury and their partners. EFT has been influenced by both systemic and attachment theory, in addition to principles suggested by Carl Rogers (1986a, 1987) to maximise empathic connections with therapy clients.

EFT proceeds by identifying negative interaction cycles that mediate conflict in romantic relationships. These cycles are characterised by both overt communication behaviours (e.g., pursuing or withdrawing from another, increasing overt distress or distancing and minimising emotional expression) and underlying attachment fears (e.g., of rejection, abandonment, being isolated and alone whilst vulnerable). Early attachment experiences are carefully assessed and then linked to relationship patterns in adulthood. The EFT therapist encourages a couple to be aware of such cycles, which in itself can have the effect of reducing conflict. However, a more critical stage follows where the couple are supported to express and respond to attachment needs in (emotionally moving) pro-nurturing positive interactions. The EFT therapist will actively work in the room to support the couple to exit out of the negative cycle and reach out to each other within a positive interaction. Yeates (2014) has suggested that EFT offers all the necessary ingredients of a social cognition rehabilitation intervention, informed by contemporary social and affective neuroscientific theory. We present here a case that illustrates the formulation of relationship distress post-brain injury through the attachment-informed observational lens of EFT and the main elements of the couples' intervention that followed.

Case Example: Carl (56) had been managing the ongoing consequences of a right acoustic neuroma (tumour) that was pushing on his right temporal cortex and cerebellum. In addition to hearing loss on his right side, Carl also struggled with attention and memory difficulties, plus initiation of complex planning. He asked for psychology input (he initially requested cognitive-behavioural therapy) to manage his developing feelings of depression and self-critical thinking. He came to the first appointment accompanied by his wife Sarah. Carl told the therapist (GY) how in the last few months he constantly felt like a failure at home, forgetting things, mishearing Sarah and not responding to her needs. When he acutely felt like a failure, he would banish himself in a cupboard/study under their stairs and make himself do memory exercises (this was described in a way that framed these tasks as a form of punishment). As Carl told GY this, he was tearful and could not hold eye-contact, his sense of shame palpable in the room. Sarah was watching him the whole time as he narrated his experiences, also tearful. She seemed to want to comfort him, but held back, unable to traverse Carl's self-imposed wall of shame. I asked Sarah what it was like for her in those moments when Carl banished himself under the stairs, to which she replied: 'I lose my husband'.

Although an individual therapy was requested by Carl, the risk was that it would become another form of self-imposed exile for Carl, another space to which he could 'sort himself out' but which would act to further minimise opportunities for the couple to increase their emotional connection with each other and indeed use this as a resource in their ongoing adaptation to the brain injury in their lives together and its consequences. GY reflected back to them that both suffered in these moments, and instead of Carl receiving individual therapy, perhaps they could consider taking this journey together and attend couples sessions. The couple was surprised at this invitation (see preceding section) but readily accepted.

The couple completed seven sessions of Emotionally Focused Couples Therapy (alongside vocational support provided within the Community Head Injury Service), with GY and a male colleague working as a co-therapy team. The first intervention session involved taking both partner's attachment histories, using interview questions based on the Couples Attachment Interview (CAI, Alexandrov, Cowan, & Cowan, 2005). Carl described how he struggled with several childhood illness, to which his father responded in a critical and abusive manner throughout (Carl was not the strong, athletic son his father wanted). Carl was bullied at school. He had married before meeting Sarah, but the relationship ended when he discovered his ex-wife had been cheating on him. He has three adult daughters from this first marriage, and he enjoys positive, close and self-enhancing contact with all of them. For her part, Sarah described how her family were close, but her mother had a neurological condition, so she spent her teenage and young adult years as a carer to her and had adopted a default-position of putting other people's needs before her own at all times from that point onwards. As a couple, Carl and Sarah had enjoyed eight years of a close relationship before the onset of the neuroma.

Also, in the first therapy session, the couple described examples of difficult moments between them. Carl narrated about a recent time when Sarah had been calling to him from upstairs, but his hearing difficulties prevented him from locating her position and accurately hearing her requested. She was mildly frustrated in the moment as a result. Carl then had a short nap, woke up an hour later and called for Sarah. He couldn't find her in the house. In the session Carl described (in a matter-of-fact way) how he panicked that Sarah had left him (she was working in the garden without his realising). GY stopped Carl at this point, wanting to deepen the emotional exploration of this moment in the story. He asked Carl: 'so in that confusing, disorientating place when you don't know where Sarah is in a given moment (a repeating experience given the hearing difficulties), the first conclusion that that you reach is that she has left you, abandoned you?'

Carl became tearful and looked at Sarah. However, at this point she looked away, starting to close down on him. "I can't believe that you could think that after all this time". GY intervened, reflecting back that this is hard for Sarah to hear, given her longstanding commitment to the relationship and love for Carl, which she so desperately needs him to take in to himself. Sarah nodded. GY then turned to Carl:

> and the reason that it is Sarah above anyone else that inadvertently triggers these fears in you, is because she is so important to you, you love her so

much, and you are terrified of that love not being in your life now, when you need it most?

Carl nodded his head vigorously, wiping his tears away from his eyes. GY maintained the pace of this emotional intensification and said: "can you tell her Carl? Can you turn to Sarah, look her in the eyes, and tell her how important she is to you?" Carl turned to Sarah and communicated movingly how he needed her so much and how the difficulties related to the tumour, and the mistakes he now frequently made, left him with a desperate fear that he would lose her. Sarah rushed to his side and they embraced lovingly, intensely.

GY used EFT techniques of evocative responding, heightening and finally choreographed an enactment to create a pro-nurturing interactional change event between the couple, hypothesised in the EFT model to deepen emotional reprocessing of attachment figures and linked to positive therapy outcomes within the EFT process research. This powerful interaction was supported in the first session and repeated in the subsequent meetings. In this way the couple were supported to progressively exit out of a negative cycle that had formed post-injury (Figure 7.1). This pattern triggered attachment fears that were established for both partners in their earlier lives and now reactivated post-injury. Uncertain of the other's needs and feelings, and sensitive to not making the other feel worse, both partners adopted attachment strategies of withdrawal, creating the withdraw–withdraw cycle in Figure 7.2. While

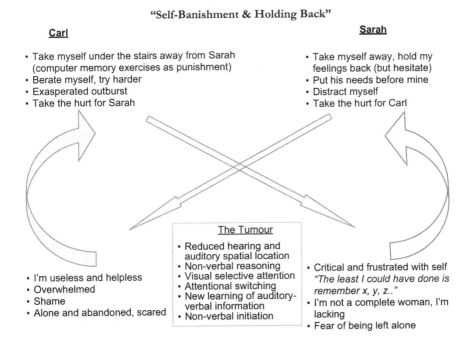

"Self-Banishment & Holding Back"

Carl

Sarah

- Take myself under the stairs away from Sarah (computer memory exercises as punishment)
- Berate myself, try harder
- Exasperated outburst
- Take the hurt for Sarah

- Take myself away, hold my feelings back (but hesitate)
- Put his needs before mine
- Distract myself
- Take the hurt for Carl

The Tumour
- Reduced hearing and auditory spatial location
- Non-verbal reasoning
- Visual selective attention
- Attentional switching
- New learning of auditory-verbal information
- Non-verbal initiation

- I'm useless and helpless
- Overwhelmed
- Shame
- Alone and abandoned, scared

- Critical and frustrated with self *"The least I could have done is remember x, y, z.."*
- I'm not a complete woman, I'm lacking
- Fear of being left alone

FIGURE 7.2 Negative Withdraw-Withdraw Cycle between Carl and Sarah

not characterised by over conflict and argument, this cycle insidiously increased disconnection and distance between Carl and Sarah, with quiet and private bit significant distress for them both.

The bulk of the intervention was conducted across six fortnightly sessions, with a two months follow-up seventh session. In this final session, both partners spontaneously moved their chairs to be close together. They had recently returned from a holiday in Rome and lovingly narrated a new story to illustrate their experienced change in their relationship. Both partners had stepped into a lift during their stay in the Italian capital but were then followed by several other people, and the lift suddenly became very crowded. They were slightly separated by the packed mass of bodies and both were a little anxious in these unfamiliar surroundings. However, Carl reached out and found Sarah's waiting hand and they both felt secure and calm. At this point an Italian lady in the lift noticed this and said: 'ah . . . amore bella!'

Conclusions

We made a case for the centrality of attachment and its disruption in the experiences of ABI survivors and their significant others, consistent with the scope of attachment theory itself. In particular we have articulated how patterns of attachment dysregulation can spread across wider levels of relationship around a survivor and in so doing exacerbate the levels of distress and disconnection for all concerned. Finally, we have proposed how a focus on emotion, relationships, distress and intra/interpersonal dysregulation could organise both specific interventions for individuals, couples and families but also a neurorehabilitation response as a whole.

This latter perspective is consistent with those studies that show quality of working alliances between TBI patients and the rehabilitation staff are related to measures of productivity after rehabilitation was completed (Prigatano et al., 1994; Klonoff, Lamb, & Henderson, 2001) and wider indices of rehabilitation outcome (Schönberger, Humle, & Teasdale, 2006a, 2006b, 2007; Schönberger, Humle, Zeeman, & Teasdale, 2006a, 2006b). Furthermore, the injury-related social cognition challenges to significant relationships noted in this chapter similarly influence therapeutic working relationships with rehabilitation clinicians to a greater extent than other domains of cognitive impairment (Schönberger et al., in press). The case for formulating the attachment dimension and its disruption at all levels of relationship and as core to the endeavour of neurorehabilitation is unequivocal.

Acknowledgements

GY would like to acknowledge the skilful therapeutic work of Dr Aonghus Ryan, his co-therapist in the EFT intervention.

References

Ahmad, T., & Yeates, G. N. (2017). *Sex & sexuality after brain injury*. UK: Headway.

Ainsworth, M. D. S. (1993). Attachments and other affectional bonds across the life cycle. In C. M. Parkes, J. Stevenson-Hinde, & P. Marris (Eds.), *Attachment across the life cycle* (pp. 33–51). New York: Routledge.

Ainsworth, M. D. S., Blehar, M. C., Waters, E., & Wall, S. (1978). *Patterns of attachment: A psychological study of the strange situation*. Hillsdale, NJ: Erlbaum.

Alexandrov, E. O., Cowan, P. A., & Cowan, C. P. (2005). Couple attachment and the quality of marital relationships: Method and concept in the validation of the new couple attachment interview and coding system. *Attachment & Human Development*, 7(2), 123–152.

Ashworth, F. (2014). Soothing the injured brain with a compassionate mind: Building the case for compassion focused therapy following acquired brain injury. *Neuro-Disability and Psychotherapy*, 2(1–2), 41–79.

Ashworth, F., Clarke, A., Jones, L., Jennings, C., & Longworth, C. (2015). An exploration of compassion focused therapy following acquired brain injury. *Psychology and Psychotherapy: Theory, Research and Practice*, 88(2), 143–162.

Ashworth, F., Gracey, F., & Gilbert, P. (2011). Compassion focused therapy after traumatic brain injury: Theoretical foundations and a case illustration. *Brain Impairment*, 12(2), 128–139.

Bar, M. (2009). Predictions in the brain: Using our past to prepare for the future. *Philosophical Transactions of the Royal Society*, 364(1521), 1179–1341.

Bechara, A., Damasio, A. R., Damasio, H., & Anderson, S. W. (1994). Insensitivity to future consequences following damage to human prefrontal cortex. *Cognition*, 50, 7–15.

Blair, R., & Cipolotti, L. (2000). Impaired social response reversal: A case of acquired sociopathy. *Brain*, 123, 1122–1141.

Blonder, L. X., Pettigrew, L. C., & Kryscio, R. J. (2012). Emotion recognition and marital satisfaction in stroke. *Journal of Clinical and Experimental Neuropsychology*, 34(6), 634–642. https://doi.org/10.1080/13803395.2012.667069

Boss, P., & Couden, B. (2002). Ambiguous loss from chronic physical illness. Journal of Clinical Psychology, 58(11), 1351–1360.

Bowen, C., Yeates, G. N., & Palmer, S. (2010). *A relational approach to rehabilitation: Thinking about relationships after brain injury*. London: Karnac Books.

Bowlby, J. (1969). *Attachment and loss. Volume I: Attachment*. New York: Basic Books.

Bowlby, J. (1973). *Attachment and loss. Volume II: Separation*. New York: Basic Books.

Bowlby, J. (1979). *Vínculos afectivos: Formación, desarrollo y pérdida*. Madrid: Morata.

Browne, C. J., & Shlosberg, E. (2006). Attachment theory, ageing and dementia: A review of the literature. *Aging and Mental Health*, 10(2), 134–142.

Butler, E. A., & Randall, A. K. (2013). Emotional coregulation in close relationships. *Emotion Review*, 5(2), 202–210.

Calkins, S. D., & Leerkes, E. M. (2004). Early attachment processes and the development of emotional self-regulation. In R. F. Baumeister & K. D. Vohs (Eds.), *Handbook of self-regulation: Research, theory, and applications* (pp. 324–339). New York: Guilford Press.

Cassidy, J. (1994). Emotion regulation: Influences of attachment relationships. *Monographs of the Society for Research in Child Development*, 59(2–3), 228–249.

Channon, S., & Crawford, S. (2000). The effects of anterior lesions on performance on a story comprehension test: Left anterior impairment on a theory of mind-type task. *Neuropsychologia*, 38, 1006–1017.

Channon, S., Pellijeff, A., & Rule, A. (2005). Social cognition after head injury: Sarcasm and theory of mind. *Brain & Language, 93,* 123–134.

Chawla, N., & Kafescioglu, N. (2012). Evidenced-based couples therapy for chronic illness: Enriching the emotional quality of relationships with emotionally-focused therapy. *Journal of Family Psychotherapy, 23*(1), 42–53.

Cheston, R., Thorne, K., Whitby, P., & Peak, J. (2007). Simulated presence therapy, attachment and separation amongst people with dementia. *Dementia, 6*(3), 442–449.

Clulow, C. (2001). *Adult attachment and couple psychotherapy: The 'secure base' in practice and research.* London: Karnac Books.

Coetzer, R. (2009). A clinical pathway including psychotherapy approaches for managing emotional difficulties after acquired brain injury. *CNS Spectrums, 14*(11), 632–638.

Coetzer, R., Yeates, G. N., Balchin, R., & Schmidt, K. (2018). I am who I am through who we are: The potential role of ubuntu in neurorehabilitation. *Panamerican Journal of Neuropsychology, 12*(2).

Crittenden, P. (1995). Attachment and psychopathology. In S. Goldberf, R. Muir, & J. Kerr (Eds.), *Attachment theory: Social, developmental and clinical aspects* (pp. 367–406). Mahweh, NJ: Analytic Press.

Crittenden, P., & Landini, A. (2011). *Assessing adult attachment: A dynamic maturational approach to discourse analysis.* New York: W.W. Norton & Company.

Daisley, A., & Webster, G. (2008). Familial brain injury: Impact on and interventions with children. In A. Tyerman & N. King (Eds.), *Psychological approaches to rehabilitation after traumatic brain injury* (pp. 475–509). Oxford: Blackwell.

Feeney, B. (2006). An attachment perspective on the interplay between intrapersonal and inter personal processes. In K. Vohs & E. Finkel (Eds.), *Self and relationships: Connecting intrapersonal and interpersonal processes.* New York: Guilford Press.

Feigelson, C. (1993). Personality death, object loss, and the uncanny. *The International Journal of Psycho-Analysis, 74*(2), 331.

Fonagy, P., Steele, M., Steele, H., Leigh, T., Kennedy, R., Mattoon, G., & Target, M. (1995). Attachment, the reflective self and borderline states: The predictive specificity of the Adult Attachment Interview and pathological emotional development. In S. Goldberg, R. Muir, & J. Kerr (Eds.), *Attachment theory: Social, developmental and clinical perspectives.* New York: The Analytic Press.

Freed, P. (2002). Meeting of the minds: Ego reintegration after traumatic brain injury. *Bulletin of the Menninger Clinic, 66*(1), 61–78.

George, C., Kaplan, N., & Main, M. (1985). *Attachment interview for adults.* Unpublished manuscript. Berkeley, CA: University of California.

Gilbert, P. (2005). *Compassion: Conceptualisations, research and use in psychotherapy.* Hove, UK: Routledge.

Gosling, J., & Oddy, M. (1999). Rearranged marriages: Marital relationships after head injury. *Brain Injury, 13,* 785–796.

Haslam, C., Holme, A., Haslam, S. A., Lyer, A., Jetten, J., & Williams, W. H. (2008). Maintaining group memberships: Social identity continuity predicts well-being after stroke. *Neuropsychological Rehabilitation, 18,* 671–691.

Hofer, M. A. (1994). Early relationships as regulators of infant physiology and behavior. *Acta Paediatrica, 83,* 9–18.

Hofer, M. A. (1994). Hidden regulators in attachment, separation, and loss. In N. A. Fox (Ed.), *The development of emotion regulation: Biological and behavioral considerations.* Monographs of the Society for Research in Child Development, Vol. 59, No. 2–3, Serial No. 240 (pp. 192–207). Chicago, IL: University of Chicago Press.

Hornak, J., Bramham, J., Rolls, E. T., Morris, R. G., O'Doherty, J., Bullock, P. R., & Polkey, C. E. (2003). Changes in emotion after circumscribed surgical lesions of the orbitofrontal and cingulate cortices. *Brain*, *126*, 1691–1712.

Johnson, S. M. (2002). *Emotionally focused couples therapy with trauma survivors: Strengthening the attachment bonds*. New York, NY: Guildford Press.

Johnson, S. (2004). *The practice of emotionally-focussed couples therapy: Creating connection*. New York: Other Press.

Klonoff, P. S., Lamb, D. G., & Henderson, S. W. (2001). Outcomes from milieu-based neurorehabilitation at up to 11 years post-discharge. *Brain Injury*, *15*(5), 413–428.

Kokkonen, T. M., Cheston, R. I., Dallos, R., & Smart, C. A. (2014). Attachment and coping of dementia care staff: The role of staff attachment style, geriatric nursing self-efficacy, and approaches to dementia in burnout. *Dementia*, *13*(4), 544–568.

Landau, J., & Hissett, J. L. (2008). Mild traumatic brain injury: Impact on identity and ambiguous loss in the family. *Family Systems and Health*, *26*(1), 69–85.

Main, M. (1995). Attachment: Overview, with implications for clinical work. In S. Goldberg, R. Muir, & J. Kerr (Eds.), *Attachment theory: Social, developmental, and clinical perspectives* (pp. 407–474). Hillsdale, NJ: Analytic Press.

Main, M., & Solomon, J. (1990). Procedures for identifying infants as disorganized/disoriented during Ainsworth Strange Situation. In M. Greenberg, D. Cicchetti, & M. Cummings (Eds.), *Attachment in the preschool years: Theory, research and intervention* (pp. 121–160). Chicago, IL: University of Chicago Press.

Maitz, E. A., & Sachs, P. R. (1995). Treating families of individuals with traumatic brain injury from a family systems perspective. *Journal of Head Trauma Rehabilitation*, *10*, 1–11.

Mauss-Clum, N., & Ryan, M. (1981). Brain injury and the family. *Journal of Neurosurgical Nursing*, *13*, 165–169.

McDonald, S., Flanagan, S., Rollins, J., & Kinch, J. (2003). TASIT: A new clinical tool for assessing social perception after traumatic brain injury. *Journal of Head Trauma Rehabilitation*, *18*, 219–238.

Miesen, B. (1992). Attachment theory and dementia. *Caregiving in Dementia: Research and Applications*, *1*, 38–56.

Miesen, B. (1993). Alzheimer's disease, the phenomenon of parent fixation and Bowlby's attachment theory. *International Journal of Geriatric Psychiatry*, *8*, 147–153.

Miesen, B. (1999). *Dementia in close-up. Understanding and caring for people with dementia*. London and New York: Routledge.

Miesen, B., & Jones, G. (1997). Psychic pain resurfacing in dementia. From new to past trauma? In L. Hunt, M. Marshall, & C. Rowlings (Eds.), *Past trauma in late life. European perspectives on therapeutic work with older people* (pp. 142–154). London: Jessica Kingsley.

Nelis, S. M., Clare, L., & Whitaker, C. J. (2014). Attachment in people with dementia and their caregivers: A systematic review. *Dementia*, *13*(6), 747–767.

Niven, K., Totterdell, P., & Holman, D. (2009). A classification of controlled interpersonal affect regulation strategies. *Emotion*, *9*(4), 498.

Oddy, M. (2001). Sexual relationships following brain injury. *Sexual Relationship Therapy*, *16*, 247–259.

Panksepp, J. (1998). *Affective neuroscience*. New York: Oxford University Press.

Perlesz, A., Kinsella, G., & Crowe, S. (2000). Psychological distress and family satisfaction following traumatic brain injury: Injured individuals and their primary, secondary, and tertiary carers. *Journal of Head Trauma Rehabilitation*, *15*, 909–929.

Pincus, D., Freeman, W., & Modell, A. (2007). Neurobiological model of perception: Considerations for transference. *Psychoanalytic Psychology*, *24*(4), 623.

Porges, S. W. (2009, April). The polyvagal theory: New insights into adaptive reactions of the autonomic nervous system. *Cleveland Clinic Journal of Medicine, 76*(Supplement 2), S86–S90.

Prigatano, G. P. (1991). Disordered mind, wounded soul: The emerging role of psychotherapy in rehabilitation after brain injury. *The Journal of Head Trauma Rehabilitation.*

Prigatano, G. P. (1999). *Principles of neuropsychological rehabilitation.* Oxford University Press.

Prigatano, G. P. (2008). Neuropsychological rehabilitation and psychodynamic psychotherapy. In J. Morgan & J. Ricker (Eds.), *Textbook of clinical neuropsychology* (pp. 985–995). New York: Taylor and Francis.

Prigatano, G. P. (2011). The importance of the patient's subjective experience in stroke rehabilitation. *Topics in Stroke Rehabilitation, 18*(1), 30–34.

Prigatano, G. P., Klonoff, P. S., O'Brien, K. P., Altman, I. M., Amin, K., Chiapello, D. . . . Mora, M. (1994). Productivity after neuropsychologically oriented milieu rehabilitation. *The Journal of Head Trauma Rehabilitation, 9*(1), 91–102.

Prigatano, G. P., & Salas, C. E. (2017). Psychodynamic psychotherapy after severe traumatic brain injury. In T. McMillan & R. Wood (Eds.), *Neurobehavioural disability and social handicap following traumatic brain injury* (pp. 189–201). New York: Psychology Press.

Rogers, C. (1986a, 1987). Reflection of feelings and transference. In H. Kirschenbaum & V. L. Henderson (Eds.), *The Carl Rogers readers (1990).* London: Constable & Robinson.

Salas, C. E. (2012). Surviving catastrophic reaction after brain injury: The use of self-regulation and self-other regulation. *Neuropsychoanalysis, 14*(1), 77–92.

Salas, C. E. (2014). Research digest. *Neuropsychoanalysis, 16*(2), 153–158.

Salas, C. E., Casassus, M., Rowlands, L., Pimm, S., & Flanagan, D. A. (2018). "Relating through sameness": A qualitative study of friendship and social isolation in chronic traumatic brain injury. *Neuropsychological Rehabilitation, 28*(7), 1161–1178.

Salas, C. E., Radovic, D., Yuen, K. S., Yeates, G. N., Castro, O., & Turnbull, O. H. (2014). "Opening an emotional dimension in me": Changes in emotional reactivity and emotion regulation in a case of executive impairment after left fronto-parietal damage. *Bulletin of the Menninger Clinic, 78*(4), 301–334.

Sander, A. M., & Struchen, M. A. (2011). Interpersonal relationships and traumatic brain injury. *The Journal of Head Trauma Rehabilitation, 26*(1), 1–3.

Schore, A. (2003). *Affect dysregulation and the disorders of the self.* New York: W.W. Norton & Company Inc.

Siegel, D. J. (1999). *The developing mind.* New York: Guilford Press.

Humle, F., & Teasdale, T. W. (2006a). The development of the therapeutic working alliance, patients' awareness and their compliance during the process of brain injury rehabilitation. *Brain Injury, 20*(4), 445–454.

Schönberger, M., Humle, F., & Teasdale, T. W. (2006b). Subjective outcome of brain injury rehabilitation in relation to the therapeutic working alliance, client compliance and awareness. *Brain Injury, 20*(12), 1271–1282.

Schönberger, M., Humle, F., & Teasdale, T. W. (2007). The relationship between client's cognitive functioning and the therapeutic working alliance in post-acute brain injury rehabilitation. *Brain Injury, 21*(8), 825–836.

Schönberger, M., Humle, F., Zeeman, P., & Teasdale, T. W. (2006a). Patient compliance in brain injury rehabilitation in relation to awareness and cognitive and physical improvement. *Neuropsychological Rehabilitation, 16*(5), 561–578.

Schönberger, M., Humle, F., Zeeman, P., & Teasdale, T. W. (2006b). Working alliance and patient compliance in brain injury rehabilitation and their relation to psychosocial outcome. *Neuropsychological Rehabilitation, 16*(3), 298–314.

Schönberger, M., Yeates, G. N., & Hobbs, P. (in press). Associations between therapeutic working alliance and social cognition in neuro-rehabilitation. *Neuropsychological Rehabilitation*.

Solms, M. (2014). A neuropsychoanalytical approach to the hard problem of consciousness. *Journal of Integrative Neuroscience, 13*(2), 173–185.

Stiell, K., & Gailey, G. (2011). Emotionally focused therapy for couples living with aphasia. In J. L. Furrow, S. M. Johnson, & B. A. Bradley (Eds), *The emotionally focused casebook* (pp. 113–140). New York, NY: Routledge.

Stiell, K., Naaman, S. C., & Lee, A. (2007). Couples and chronic illness: An attachment perspective and emotionally-focused interventions. *Journal of Systemic Therapies, 26*, 59–74.

Yeates, G. N. (2009). Working with families in neuropsychological rehabilitation. In B. A. Wilson, F. Gracey, J. J. Evans, & A. Bateman (Eds.), *Neuropsychological rehabilitation: Theory, models, therapy & outcome*. Cambridge: Cambridge University Press.

Yeates, G. N. (2013). Towards the neuropsychological foundations of couples therapy following Acquired Brain Injury (ABI): A review of empirical evidence and relevant concepts. *Neuro-disability and Psychotherapy, 1*(1), 108–150.

Yeates, G. N. (2014). Social cognition interventions in neuro-rehabilitation: An overview. *Advances in Clinical Neuroscience & Rehabilitation, 14*(2), 12–13.

Yeates, G. N. (in press). The use of attachment theory to inform psycho-sexual couples work in neuro-rehabilitation. *Brain Injury Professional*.

Yeates, G. N., Edwards, A., Murray, C., Creamer, N., & Mahadevan, M. (2013). The use of Emotionally-Focused Couples Therapy (EFT) for survivors of acquired brain injury with social cognition and executive functioning impairments and their partners: A case series analysis. *Neuro-Disability & Psychotherapy, 1*(2), 152–189.

Yeates, G. N., Gracey, F., & Mcgrath, J. C. (2008). A biopsychosocial deconstruction of "personality change" following acquired brain injury. *Neuropsychological Rehabilitation, 18*(5–6), 566–589.

Yeates, G. N., Rowberry, M., Dunne, S., Goshawk, M., Mahadevan, M., Tyerman, R. . . . Tyerman, A. (2016). Social cognition and executive functioning predictors of supervisors' appraisal of interpersonal behaviour in the workplace following acquired brain injury. *NeuroRehabilitation, 38*(3), 299–310. https://doi.org/10.3233/NRE-161321

Zaki, J., & Williams, W. C. (2013). Interpersonal emotion regulation. *Emotion, 13*(5), 803.

8

PUTTING CONVERSATIONS CENTRE STAGE

Systemic working in acquired brain injury contexts

Gavin Newby, Siobhan Palmer, Ndidi Boakye, Jo Johnson and Richard Maddicks

Introduction

Writing about systemic thinking is often a 'collaborative exchange of voices', as personally described by Hoffman in her engaging text describing the history and development of family therapy (Hoffman, 1993). This chapter has been written as a reflective conversation between the authors. We discuss definitions of systemic work alongside how we each use systemic techniques with individuals and families affected by brain injury. We invite the reader to adopt this approach to thinking about how relationship dynamics within and between families and professional systems can influence the definition and treatment of acquired problems and ultimately the outcomes in neurorehabilitation. The conversation contains practical examples and a case example.

An orientating perspective from Gavin Newby

Actually it started with a conversation on a beach. Well two beaches to be precise – Hove, Sussex and Mossyard, Dumfriesshire. Siobhan and I had been approached to write a chapter on family and systemic therapy in ABI. To be honest, we had put it off a bit and quickly the main narrative was: 'Have you got time to write this? No, have you? We're so busy. How are we going to do this?' However, systemic and family are kindly and creative mistresses. Despite my son repeating 'Daddy who are you talking to? What's an article and why can't you do it?', even just the momentary adoption of a systemic mindset caused a dim and distant memory to surface. Why not use systemic therapy ideas to help us? In a delightful phrase, Siobhan described it being 'okay to have an orchestra of systemic voices within the one chapter'. In 2004, I wrote an article that essentially emerged from the interchange of emails between facilitators of a narrative group in a neurorehabilitation centre in Aylesbury, UK (Newby, Bushell, Cotter, &

Nangle, 2004). We had become stuck in our ideas of how to process the group dynamics and hit upon using the trading of emails as a medium to free up our thinking. A quote from the original article hopefully elucidates our thinking at the time:

> Unlike direct conversation, dialogues emerge piece by piece. Responses are delayed by the speed of the correspondents' typing . . . and where the receiver opens the email. . . . These delays interact with the mental state of the receiver and the further mental processing that inevitably occurs through the review of the typed response. . . . Because such dialogues have a narrative life of their own and can nail down thoughts and reflections, email can be invaluable in making ephemeral concepts concrete.
>
> *(Newby et al., 2004, p. 29)*

I have developed these ideas more fully with Rudi Coetzer in two articles from 2013. I tie the ideas specifically to Orlinsky and Howard's Generic Model of Psychotherapy (1986, 1995), who proposed that emails and even SMS text messaging can augment and extend psychotherapeutic effect beyond the consultation room. Both emails and texts are suggested to be convenient, portable, accessible, normal and universal media that can allow for cognitive reflection, the co-construction and re-authoring of therapeutic narratives (Newby & Coetzer, 2013a). In a safe therapeutic context, emails and texts can aid contracting, collaboration, self-awareness, heighten session impacts and waymark the phases of treatment (Newby & Coetzer, 2013b). They contended that:

> text and email interactions could lead to third order reflexivity. Third order reflection recognises that people develop their understandings of themselves through an ongoing language and experiential interaction between themselves, their immediate family and social contexts and the wider world of cultures and subcultures (which, in this day-and-age will also include social media such as Facebook and Twitter). In a therapeutic context, this means that new therapeutic insights develop through repeated cycles of therapist(s) and client(s) re-sharing and re-reflecting on the interactions evident both in the therapy room and outside. There is an important role of all parties (including therapists) abrogating the expert/having all the answers, recognising their own biases and contexts and the ways that they influence what you perceive. In this way, texts and emails can allow therapists and clients to develop shared solutions that are more likely to be effective and long-lasting. Such a mode of thinking is naturally fostered by the repeating cycles of composing and reflecting on reflections inherent in text and email interchanges. The cycles are out with the immediacy and social noise of direct face-face communication and are punctuated by time delays that aid reflection and give oxygen to being able to stand apart and try out new ideas.
>
> *(Newby & Coetzer, 2013b, p. 217)*

Quite apart from the epistemological, theoretical and therapeutic benefits of this approach, email interchange is convenient, speedy and in the moment. So . . . what's good enough for therapeutic work is surely plenty good enough for writing an article.

Narrative therapy is a gift that keeps on giving. In the spirit of our aims and title, we want this article to be a doable thing, a systemic thing and true to its epistemological roots.

It is important to establish what systemic therapy is and is not. Firstly, there is no one single systemic or family therapy. Hopefully without mixing metaphors, the Systemic approach is truly a 'family' of interlinked therapies and techniques. They are linked by the idea that you can 'understand and address an individual's difficulties within the context of their relationships' (Weatherhead et al., 2013). This means that the therapeutic focus is on understanding what a defined system is, its communication patterns, belief systems, the mutual influence of the people within the system and the wider cultural context. Pointing these influences and processes out and finding ways to positively change them forms the bases for systemic interventions. There is more than one way to skin a cat. As such there are a plethora of important and valid schools of thought and practice that have evolved from the 1950s ranging from the homeostatic 'engineering'-type systems espoused by Bateson and colleagues to Minuchin's Structural Family Therapy and the Milan Model. From the 1980s onwards, the field exploded with a several approaches and conceptual frameworks like cybernetics, social constructionism, narrative therapy and brief solution-focused therapy, to name a few. It is way beyond the scope of this chapter to explore all of these; it would be easy to drown in a morass of models, techniques, teams and complex theoretical positions, all clothed in a sometimes impenetrable language. However, I would warmly direct the interested reader towards Rudi Dallos and Ros Draper's excellent and lucid textbook *An Introduction to Family Therapy: Systemic Theory and Practice* (2015).

For me, family therapy, or systemic therapy, has never been about working with teams and two-way mirrors (often the focus of traditional systemic interventions). It's always been more about having an ever open systemic ear, thinking about the system in all my work and how the ideas could be practically embedded in ordinary, routine and everyday work situations. Looking at the narrative of my published work in this area there is a consistent theme of working to your area and available time. In 2003, working with older adults, it was about creating an organisational entity that would be recognised by managers (Newby & Thorn, 2003). A clinic was born. Seeds were sewn with short, regular workshops on learning practical techniques like circular questioning. A systemic 'win' was hearing Community Psychiatric Nurses (CPNs) routinely use them with clients and teach the technique to nursing students. There was a little bit of set piece therapy with its organisational marque of National Health Service (NHS) recognition, outcome measures and a nice leaflet to give to clients, families, professionals and commissioners. All of these initiatives were great for centring and cementing practice, but they were only the tip of the systemic iceberg. Over the years GN has developed in room supervision in casework and supervision and opportunistic observer witness group initiatives with colleagues such as Ste Weatherhead and Bernie Walsh (e.g., Bowen et al., 2009; Weatherhead & Newby, 2011). Over the years I have felt less need to name the systemic elephant in the room. It's gone into the jungle and gone native. By this I mean it has become so ingrained that I almost forget I'm doing it.

At this point whilst I feel impelled to say: don't get over-focused on process and organisations (important but . . .). It's important to put the ABI meat in the sandwich. With ABI and family stuff it's important to look at adaptations.

Again, I would draw from Rudi Coetzer (Weatherhead et al., 2013):

> Each clinical area has its own "do's and don'ts", or particular characteristics which tend to influence practice. Working psychotherapeutically with clients who have a brain injury commonly presents practitioners with many unique challenges. Judd and Wilson (2005), in a qualitative study, reported some of the obstacles encountered by clinicians during psychotherapy interventions for clients with acquired brain injury. According to these authors, some of the more frequent practitioner-reported difficulties included memory problems and negative reactions (Judd & Wilson, 2005). These and other difficulties common to many forms of acquired brain injury, including poor attention, distractibility, impairment of executive control function, poor insight, apathy, and language difficulties often require the practitioner to be creative in adapting processes and strategies.
>
> Generic therapy skills are just as important in brain injury rehabilitation work, but some specific adaptations might be useful with this population, as listed below.
>
> - Practitioners need to be aware of the pace in sessions:
>   - go slowly
>   - focus on the present while maintaining an understanding of the contribution of the person's individual history.
> - Help clients to gain perspective on reality, and try to assist them to derive a sense of meaning or purpose after brain injury.
> - Be honest and empathic with patients (adapted from Prigatano, 1999).
>
> *(pp. 67–68, Op Cit.)*

Turning this towards the world of systemic work, communicating the rationale, purpose of any formal family therapy with mirrors, in-room supervision, etc., or other classic features of formal systemic therapy (see Vetere & Dallos, 2003) for further description) would need to be very carefully thought out. Family and systemic therapy has a reputation (not least to professionals) of being clothed in obscure language and ideas. In the past, I have introduced the prospect of such work well in advance and over a number of sessions, ensured a family member is party to the early discussions (so that they can help reinforce what was said, correct any misinterpretations that lead to fears of what was about to happen and to act as an advocate for the brain injured client as and when they have questions in and out of sessions) and backed up the discussions with a tailor written document finalising what they had agreed to. With clients that I have been emailing or texting with, I have used these avenues to back up the information as well as audio recordings via smartphones and dictaphones. You might want to negotiate the use of video recordings of some sort – both as a third order reflective tool for all involved but also as a straightforward memory reminder of what had happened. Don't forget to summarise frequently during the session, watch out for the client becoming overloaded (e.g., they stop responding, appear distracted and fidgety or, indeed, become negative and oppositional) and have frequent breaks. Also, use whatever strategies you've agreed to back up the main take home messages. As regards managing the family dynamics, it can be really important to identify a member of the team, or family, who will act as an advocate during the session and will be a mentor for processing the issues discussed during breaks and after the session. Finally, don't forget to do that ending letter, with as much information as helps aid recall without being too wordy. For a more detailed exposition on specific adaptations to systemic working in ABI, please see Chapter 9 pp. 187–230 in Bowen, Yeates, and Palmer (2010).

Also, just to change tack here, we'd also like to introduce the idea of an ABI systemic competence model. I'm not sure that all and every systemic practitioner and intervention needs to be totally submersed in ABI knowledge – not least if the ABI is relatively mild or moderate and the issues are not necessarily ABI-centric, and the client can cope (whatever that means), but as the practitioner you need to have some understanding.

In recent times, there have been excellent moves in the UK to develop competency frameworks to guide professional and therapeutic practice. Happily there are such frameworks for both Clinical Neuropsychology (of which ABI is a major area) and Systemic Therapy. These are contained in the following links:

www.bps.org.uk/system/files/Public%20files/required_competences_for_clinical_neuropsychology.pdf

www.ucl.ac.uk/pals/research/clinical-educational-and-health-psychology/research-groups/core/competence-frameworks-1

Adaptations or actually simplifications would include having an understanding of ABI and its consequences for therapy and how you communicate and practice the therapy.

I had the not exactly startling insight when out running one night that we all (me included) seem a little put off committing to writing this chapter. As my mind cleared (one of the main reasons for running these days), I immediately settled upon whether it was some sort of burden of complexity that was holding us back. It's maybe a multifaceted complex burden in that (1) the subject matter can be complex to write given its myriad of terms and often impenetrable engineering-type language, girding one's loins to write it up is an often daunting prospect, particularly if you want (or think you want) the 'difficult to read' badge of systemic respectability; (2) writing an academic chapter per se takes time, is peer reviewed and is a very public way of testing whether one's ideas make the professional mark; (3) it doesn't half make you wonder, thinking about writing up, whether you are a true believer (I know when I reflect on my practice, I'm very much an eclectic practitioner, out of necessity and belief, and my therapeutic modus operandi is a mish-mash, hopefully considered, flexible and appropriate, of systemic, personal construct, CBT, behavioural ideas with a smidgeon of mindfulness.

My attempted answer to this is to be mindful, if you are allowed to in a systemic enterprise. In a nutshell, if the need we have at the moment is primarily 'to make this doable' then surely we can all reflect on how we make our practice doable. Not many of us work in reflecting teams and have two-way mirrors, etc. Rather, and we know we're mixing two therapeutic modes here, we adopt a systemic orientation, way of thinking and mindset. We apply systemic thinking in small, but effective, ways in our clinical lives. It's often in the small things. Rudi Coetzer, Ste Weatherhead and I have previously written about how to maintain your Continuing Professional Development (CPD). CPD is a professional yardstick of competence, being up to date and a good enough practitioner. Working with ABI, you come into contact with a plethora of interconnecting fields and disciplines that range from psychology per se, to its applied forms of clinical, neuropsychological, educational and occupational, to neuroscience, to medicine, to psychotherapies and beyond. Each of these fields have knowledge bases and practices that expand at an exponential rate. How on earth can you keep up? Well you can't, not completely anyway. You can only adopt our good old friend Winnicott's maxim, to be 'Good Enough'. To be good enough in Rudi's, Ste's and my opinion does include going to conferences and meetings. But in this financially restricted time, it's just not possible to go to all the conferences you could. Anyway, just think of the time it would take. No, rather the vast majority of being good enough is about the small everyday things you can do – reflect on a case, talk in supervision, read a chapter of a book, read an article, reflect on what a client did or did not do. It all adds up. For a more detailed discussion of this, please refer to Newby and Coetzer (2012), Newby and Weatherhead (2013).

As previously discussed, hopefully, an email interchange reduces the burden but allows for small things to become an orchestra of bigger, considered and insightful things.

Siobhan Palmer takes the mic: systemic therapy in day-to-day work

Sitting in my flat listening to the sound of the February sea, imagining runners going back and to along the seafront, clearing their mind and allowing ideas to flow, much as Gavin describes earlier, I wonder why I am sitting inside with a cluttered mind. I reread the narratives outlined earlier and bounce thoughts about 'what is systemic working in ABI' . . . can we be systemic and use mindfulness' (Kabat-Zinn, 1990). When is a mishmash still a helpful intervention and when is it an unboundaried piece of thinking that should perhaps not be given public airtime? Gradually I begin to bounce these ideas about in my mind with a lighter heart because in my view, systemic working is about seeing the whole system, the whole beautiful panoramic view. This is preferable to a 'still shot' because we receive richer information from a fluid, moving model of interacting relationships, which includes all the mishmash of real life, including the uncertainty of 'am I doing it right?' With the ability to reflect on ourselves, observe our own behaviour and comment on it in the context of everything else (or everyone else, such as is and will be, within this chapter) we begin to make links and find a way forward. By extrapolation, integrating models to some extent could still be systemic (systemic, with a small 's'), provided we have an awareness that we are doing this. We hold in mind that ultimately our work is focused on 'looking out' to how the family, environmental or professional systems are influencing our client's day-to-day experience and ability to function . . . as well as looking back in again to how the client's level of function and neurodisability is potentially influencing the system and understanding the reciprocal nature of these relationships. Ping out, pong back in again . . . ping pong and ping again as we look through different lens (different perspectives). Using visual metaphor helps me to use a new lens and move forward. The reason for my stickiness in commencing this writing is similar to those Gavin described previously, particularly because maybe in this blurring of approaches I could be criticised for doing it 'wrong'. Many of my colleagues have described this in our peer supervision sessions; the professional anxiety that we're doing it wrong. There appears to be, in so many of us, a sense of pre-emptive shame about not using sufficiently 'textbook' examples of therapy, that we are reluctant to write about the real clinical work that we do. For this reason, perhaps reflective chapters such as this are important in providing a professional narrative about creatively, flexibility and merging of models, which is what clinical psychologists are equipped to do. Perhaps in another world people should sing from the rooftops about having the strength to draw on multiple ideas whilst still holding in mind the multi system complexity of our client's experience . . . but, stop Siobhan! What's the goal? Using helpful ideas from goal management training (Levine et al., 2011), I notice I have gone way off track. Stop. Think. Breathe. I'll ground myself in something practical.

Day to day, my work with adults with brain injury requires as much reflection on family or support team process as it does on the needs of the individual with brain injury. Whilst it is fundamental to working in ABI that clinical neuropsychologists have an understanding of the interaction of cognition and emotion (WHO biopsychosocial model (Engel, 1980; Borrell-Carrió, Suchman & Epstein, 2004) and are familiar with the types of subtle but significant difficulties with reasoning, emotional processing and memory (to name some) classically observed in individuals with ABI, it appears to be increasingly important to be able to guide and support a team through the emotional undulations that they themselves will experience and to provide a space for reflecting on this. I draw on basic behaviour principles (such as described by Wood & Alderman, 2011); teams avoiding use of clinical behaviour management guidelines for fear of causing agitation in the client is a form of negative reinforcement for the team (i.e., avoiding the discomfort of withdrawing attention or giving feedback) and positive reinforcement of agitated behaviour for the individual client with ABI. Whilst this is behavioural, it is also systemic ('with a little s') because work with the whole team to have a conversation about motivators for their behaviour will help reduce avoidance, which will often in turn help the individual with ABI to modify their behaviour and potentially underpin the rehabilitation outcome. Progress achieved by looking at the micro details within communication, then the wider picture and back again: the ping pong of reflection again. This is a small example, and there are many more out there. In addition to the principles of reinforcement, we can take many ideas from behaviour therapy and apply them to team working; development of clear behavioural contracts enables communication and helps the multidisciplinary team to name the problem using the same language (Betteridge, Cotterill, & Murphy, 2017). When you've done the therapeutic work resulting in the client naming their goal, then sharing their name for the goal/target behaviour is important. Using the same language can prevent the stuckness of each team member tackling an issue in a different way and using valuable time repeating discussions about a sensitive issue with a client. Where the whole team agrees about the issue but the client has memory impairment, the behaviour guidelines/shared language means the team can quickly reengage the client in the conversation if needed.

As part of clinical supervision with a systemic practitioner, I spent time reflecting on how to comment on the 'elephant in the room' (for example, the often unspoken relationship tensions in a group or family system). The less it is spoken about the bigger it becomes, and if the system does not name the elephant sometimes it grows so big that it no longer fits in the room with the family . . . it can become so large that it gets stuck in the corridor outside, a sort of systemic avoidance of talking about the problem. This metaphor works well for the unspoken narratives that we begin to uncover within families or group dynamics that contribute to fragmented interventions, inconsistent responses, splitting within relationships and restrictions on interdisciplinary working or coordinated family support efforts. Sometimes, bringing the family into the shared therapy space (if not directly in a family meeting, then indirectly possibly by email, letter or a series of individual conversations) creates the opportunity to tentatively name the elephant so it can no longer be completely avoided. Using systemic questioning (Selvini, Boscolo, Cecchin, & Prata, 1980) to begin to notice and name the elephant ('the tension') begins a process of problem solving where the family can ally against the tension ('the problem'), and in so doing they change their relationship with it.

In many ways, talking of our professional anxieties is a little like naming the elephant. Despite my professional fear of being discovered as somehow fraudulent, for only talking about big elephants, beaches and panoramic pictures, it is wonderful to engage in conversations with systemically minded colleagues about complexities in systems and the narratives we co-construct about our own professional identities; to reflect on a recent assessment or to have those conversations that start with 'I don't really know why, but it's on my mind and I feel I'm missing something . . .'. We can become very solution focused as neuropsychologists, holding risk and responsibility, and some avoidance can begin to creep in if we think we might have it wrong, but invariably these conversations open up avenues of questioning and thinking in an uplifting (and clinically helpful) way. Systemic thinking is indeed a kind mistress; to me it is about talking about the entirety of the information available to us about the case; it allows us to draw on our intuition and propose the hypothesis that we 'dare not say'.

Looking back on my publications and presentations to date, my emphasis has been on relationships between two people, a family, or within teams . . . thinking about where communication gets 'stuck' ultimately bringing the whole thing to a standstill. In that moment of standing still, thoughts about inadequacy or frustration pop up and become toxic, making the elephant bigger and pushing it further down the corridor. In couples work, this stuckness presents when each party assumes the other has taken a defensive or critical position. Triangulating the conversation through a therapist helps to unstick (by way of reframe) and breathe life back into the communication again (Carr, 2012). Really slowing down the communication to look at tiny 'micro' behaviours within critical interactions (a helpful merge with Emotion Focused Couples Therapy; Johnson, Greenberg, & Leslie, 1987), I have found helpful in supporting clients with ABI and their family members to find concrete real life examples of where communication goes awry or becomes distorted, and it helps create a new narrative. Reframing and refocusing the spotlight on a different part of the problem breathes life into our natural curiosity and questioning (Hoffman, 1993), and in time it can provide concrete examples of how communication can be repaired. Bringing in new voices can shift and energise the narrative completely. Bringing in time: the past and the future as well as the now. What about new relationships, friends and social connections? How do we maintain a 'normal level' of social connection for our clients whilst living in residential settings? What was 'normal' for each client in the past? We write about these patterns in our book about relationships after brain injury (Bowen, Yeates, & Palmer, 2010) and in a more recent consideration of how friendship formation post-injury can become tangled up in the complexities of risk and social vulnerability (Palmer & Herbert, 2016).

A stuckness can similarly be seen in meetings, especially where different 'layers' of professionals are in attendance alongside family members and the individual with brain injury. The multiplicity of voices multiplies opportunities for complexity and also for the team to avoid it, meanwhile busying themselves with other tasks. I am increasingly aware of the potential for certain voices to be silenced in complex cases and the dominant voice to be that of the thing which can be solved using practical, measurable interventions. We know from early research that the most distressing sequalae after brain injury is not the physical limitations but changes in behaviour and communication (Thomsen, 1992; Klonoff, Lamb, & Henderson, 2001); it is no coincidence that these are the problems most often silenced. Systemic frameworks provide us with a way of commenting on process and asking new questions to help us see and work within the whole panorama.

Questions are the breath of life

In life and work it is often extremely difficult to keep focused on a project that involves tending to it regularly, laying a loving eye on it, keeping at the forefront of your mind and reflecting and shaping as you go along. It takes single-mindedness on the part of the authors. However, with this chapter, as in life and work, business and other things intruded for a long time. Over 18 months in fact. Occasionally Gavin would notice its strapline popping out of its Dropbox folder, imploring him to open it up. He would, occasionally, but then there'd be another phone call, email or text. The creative juices ran dry and we ground to a halt. Then, out of the blue, our forbearing editor gently, but firmly, asked when we'd be submitting our chapter. He kindly set us a six- week deadline to sharpen our minds.

We emailed; we spoke. We were stuck. Where to go with what we have? We remained determined to stay true to our original thoughts – write an accessible systemic chapter in a systemic way. So what do you do when you're stuck with a system? You call on other voices of course! In anticipation Siobhan had already thought of three excellent and enthusiastic proponents of practical and doable systemic working – Richard Maddicks, Ndidi Boakye and Jo Johnson.

Let's Question Our Way Out

Richard, what does systemic mean to you?
Its where we come from and our stage of professional development that forms me.

It has been suggested that the collective pronoun for psychologists should be 'a disagreement', although it wasn't until my clinical training in the UK that I became aware of the extent of the tribalism. The psychodynamic (Howard, 2011; McWilliams, 2004; Rockland, 1989) influences of the Salomons doctoral training meant that my exposure to tweedy, beardy men peddling their transference and Malanian triangles (Malan, 1995) was noticeably greater than many of my peers. Meanwhile, my 'too cool for school' metropolitan contemporaries wore their glossy, new CBT skills (Hawton, Salkovskis, Kirk, & Clark, 1994) with a somewhat smug, bulging evidence base certainty. Arguably, this conflict between the role of the clinical psychologist as a researcher/diagnostician and psychotherapist characterised the post-war development of the profession in the UK, the resulting, rhetorical, 'scientist-practitioner' model (a good, old fashioned, British compromise?), symbiotic with the new, 'pragmatic' National Health Service (Pilgrim & Treacher, 1992).

Yet, one function of clinical training is to find your own way. For me it was a chastening three-year graded exposure programme, building my capacity to tolerate uncertainty and the messy reality of people's distress and disease. My own personal history of parental separation as an adolescent seemed to make the messiness more compelling, and from all of this emerged several 'realities' that I keep with me:

- the health of the individual is more often than not interdependent with the health of their family;
- families are like kaleidoscopes. They often incorporate change beautifully and can often be remade through their members' shared histories such that possibilities are unpredictable and almost infinite;
- when we work with families we fleetingly become a piece of the kaleidoscope, like a website 'cookie' the family is asked to accept for long enough to hopefully help make sense of their new shapes and patterns.

Ndidi, you lead peer supervision meetings using systemic techniques and formulate complex team/ client dynamics using systemic ideas. What do you think about what we have been saying? What do systemic ideas help you with in your practice, and how do you 'translate' the complexity of systemic theory into doable things?

The person as therapist

When I was asked to contribute to this chapter, I remember initially feeling quite elated. This was at the thought of being considered remotely systemic (with a small 's') to contribute to a conversation on working systemically in brain injury. This was quickly replaced with some anxiety and questions such as what does it mean to be systemic and how does one begin to put that into writing?

Gavin and Siobhan have written quite eloquently about the challenges of how to make systemic practices 'do able' and how some of this may be about recognising the small ways in which we are already doing this in our clinical work. This may involve the use of emails, tape recording, video recordings or even a relative to extend the therapeutic effect. But how do we do this whilst ensuring we remain true to our systemic roots? Siobhan and Gavin raised the issue of ensuring we stay up to date with systemic practices by being mindful; this may be as simple as reflecting on a piece of work and opening up other avenues for exploration. It may be reading a systemic chapter and discussing this. The ease with which we could maintain our systemic competencies makes it 'do able' and allows us to apply these principles to our work without fear of being found wanting. However, as we develop our clinical abilities, naturally we acquire more responsibilities and that includes the supervision space. How do we adapt the supervision space to include a systemic lens? To introduce more ideas which can drive clinical decisions making? Do systemic ideas allow us to explore topics which may be challenging clinically, such as race and spirituality? If so how? How can we make exploration of these topics 'do able' also?

I am a black female of Nigerian heritage born in the UK and working as a neuropsychologist in a rehabilitation setting. In exploring positioning and reflexivity, I am writing in the first person, which enables me to take a position that acknowledges my reflexive stance. It also allows me to explore the multiple influences that impact my thinking and the positions I take in my professional setting. I am a neuropsychologist working across multiple settings, i.e., inpatient, outpatient and community. These settings bring me into varied domains, including interpersonal therapy with patients, consultations with members of the MDT, supervision and management. Furthermore, I am regularly asked to facilitate conversations around issues that arise in clinical practice.

I would describe myself as a clinical neuropsychologist with a heavy emphasis on the clinical. This is because throughout my professional training I was mindful that the field of neuropsychology was seen as for the 'intellectual' psychologist, the one interested in figures and in the complexity of the brain. However, I have never felt that I fit into that world. Indeed, on paper I meet all the requirements, but in reality I have always felt that neuropsychology is more than the brain and therefore more than the complex interpretation of statistics. After all, the brain is attached to a head, the head to a body, and the body is occupied by a mind that moves in and out of different contextual settings. These contextual settings give rise to the visible-invisible and the voice-unvoiced matrices in which we all occupy described by Burnham (2013) as the social GGRRAAACCEEESSS. This term has come to represent differences in beliefs, power and lifestyle, which we might pay attention to in therapy and in supervision. It includes gender, geography, race, religion, age, ability, appearance, class, culture, ethnicity, education, employment, sexuality, sexual orientation and spirituality. The sequelae of brain injury includes cognitive impairments, emotional and behavioural difficulties, physical disabilities and many other challenges, not least family breakdown and social isolation (Wood, Liossi, & Wood, 2005). It is imperative for me, therefore, as a neuropsychologist, to look beyond the brain and the individual and consider the systems people are occupying. The ability to draw on systemic principles in my everyday work enables me to do this.

As a black Christian woman in a largely white, secular dominated profession, I approach the topic of difference with caution, and I am painfully aware of the risk I take (even now in writing) in discussing this topic. This may be influenced by my relationship with the very visible difference I am confronted with on a daily basis: race. At work, I am ever mindful of the discomfort race can evoke in my ethnic majority colleagues. This may be manifested in an all too familiar silence, which can follow when race comes up therapeutically, in professional peer context or indeed even in the supervision space. I am mindful of my own reaction to race, including the (necessary) burden to invite others to discuss or notice 'the other'. However, I am driven by the fact that central to one's identity and sense of self is the different contexts that people have to navigate in life and the meaning one draws from this. This complex process is described well by Pearce and Cronen (1980)'s Coordinated Management of Meaning (CMM) model. When applying this systemic principle one has to hold in mind that when individuals are interacting socially, such as in a therapy space, they are collectively constructing the meaning of their conversation. However, both individuals are also comprised of an interpersonal system, which helps explain their actions and reactions. Therefore, it is important to me as a psychologist and supervisor that in the supervision space we consider the following questions: What are we shining a spotlight to in our work and why? Why are some areas left in the dark and how might we begin to hold a light to it?

Being a black Christian psychologist means that I am ever mindful of difference, mostly of how different I might be to my professional peers, how I enunciate and how I am perceived by my ethnic majority colleagues-particularly peers. Do they think I'm being 'aggressive' if I am too passionate about a subject matter? These questions come from a lifetime of 'being told' in the workplace that I'm different. Starting from conversations about my name, to how I live my life to my communication style. As a result I find myself sensitive to various things such as the anglicising of patient names, particularly those from minority backgrounds, thinking about cultural expressions of distress and raising that with the MDT, thinking about other models of healing which also bring about change and being mindful that there are alternative to the mind body dichotomy. That there are other views that humans are spirit, soul and body. At times it feels exciting and a privilege to be in a position where I can make a difference; other times it feels scary, that lone voice amongst the deadly silence. I am left wondering what the repercussions would be. However, sometimes it leads to a different clinical decision (i.e., offering a patient psychotherapy for adjustment difficulties rather than treating 'the anger' as a challenging behaviour); a small win, reminding me that my contribution to the profession can make a difference and change the course of a patient's relationship to help.

Perhaps this is why I am drawn intuitively to systemic practices. It just makes the process of exploration, which is daunting, easier. For example, although initially starting out as a theory, the social GGRRAAACCEEESSS has been as integrated in systemic practices as a tool. Primarily, this tool has been used as a way of developing cultural competencies in both the therapy and supervision space (Jones & Reeve, 2014). I am able to use this tool and the CMM in my supervision space to raise the topic of difference. It enables me to support my supervisees to ask a different question and therefore allow new information or hypotheses to the therapy space.

> Metaphor is argued to be a fundamental mechanism that allows us to use what we know about our physical and social experience to provide understanding in a wide range of other areas.
>
> *(Lakoff & Johnson, 1980)*

I like to describe clinical psychology training as being taught to play an instrument, and at the end of training you will be able to play. However, the ability to move a person from one emotional state to the next requires fine tuning, awareness of timing and mindfulness of the audience at hand; that is the art. My rationale for using this particular metaphor of playing an instrument is that as a musician you have to be engaged in the process. You are intertwined with your instrument in order to make music; it needs your hands, your mind and your mouth. This metaphor helps to provide a framework to consider what one brings into the therapy space as a psychologist, e.g., the mind, visible-invisible differences and how these factors intertwine. My role as a supervisor is therefore to develop the art in those in my supervision space.

Whether facilitating discussions about clinical issues or with my supervisees, I invite those in my supervision space to begin to discuss and engage in conversations about difference, to notice where the spotlights are, where they are not, and to have a language to describe the processes influencing this. In different moments of the conversations there are multiple personal and professional influencing contexts and a reflection on ones' cultural influences and biases at play. To discuss this openly requires the creation of a safe space, by taking risks myself and by discussing my own position and highlighting the idea that there are multiple hypotheses. I highlight the notion that a position of 'both and' allows the creation of further solutions that may facilitate clinical decision making. Barry Mason introduced the term 'safe uncertainty' and stressed its place in working systemic work. He stressed that without uncertainty being permissible, curiosity closes down, making any subsequent deep understanding of a family's difficulty unlikely. The concept of 'safe uncertainty' (Mason, 1993) is useful here in staying with the position of 'both and'. It posits that as humans, when we are not mindful of our reactions, we confuse certainty with safety, assuming that the more certain we are the safer the position. However, this is an unrealistic space, leading to a more defensive position, e.g., blocking other possibilities. As we become more aware of our unconscious biases it enables us to work towards a position of safe uncertainty – opening up a more realistic space that facilitates exploration and learning, albeit uncomfortable.

Another way of working systemically that I really enjoy is the use of reflective teams for complex formulations or case discussions. In my experience, using a systemic frame to set this up helps to create a safe and structured group setting where staff can be open about their work. The systemic frame aims to increase the capacity of staff to think from multiple perspectives and to be mindful that there are multiple 'truths'. It also seeks to improve formulation through the generation of multiple hypotheses about the causes of patient distress as well as increasing staff empathy. The use of a systemic frame draws on diverse life experiences and highlights potential dynamic issues that 'crop up' in clinical work. This includes emotional responses in relationships with patients and what one does with that. For example, what clinical decisions can take place if you like or dislike a patient/relative/carer? This increases staff understanding of patients and their families and makes MDT formulations easier. It is particularly important, as there are multiple disciplines, all using different approaches and coming from different training backgrounds. The systemic frame allows the MDT to access other approaches and experiences. Staff often report that they feel better after a reflective session. Reasons offered include feeling reassured that others share a similar experience. This helps to improve morale and can reduce staff burn out.

I have discussed the multiple systemic principles and therefore positions one can hold in the supervision space. A holding of these positions in the supervision space facilitates a greater awareness of the uniqueness of the otherness of people and allows for a therapeutic positioning, which is an important contribution to the art of therapeutic interaction.

So, coming back to the question of 'how do we make systemic work doable in neuro settings?', I believe that systemic formulation and practices are absolutely doable in a neuro setting. Furthermore, it doesn't always need adaptation because – whilst it might need adapting for individual patients – we're not just thinking about the patients and their systems, but other systems at play, i.e., our professional systems.

Narratives and dominant discourses about patient and their difficulties can be opened up in supervision and team meetings by using a bit of curiosity. This in itself can be a powerful intervention for the patient directly influencing their care – a big, doable, systemic win. My own experience of difference perhaps positions me and helps me to ask these sorts of questions and challenge the dominant narratives to open up dialogues and develop other hypotheses about a patient and their problems, moving away from medical reductionist definitions. It is a powerful tool to use in neuro settings, although probably one which (to me) feels more like a way of being than a specific tool or set of questions.

> **So, let's explore this a bit more. Jo, if our own family influences our ways of relating to families, what's it like for you working with families . . . as part of the wider neuropsychology family?**

I am who I am, no apologies. My energy comes from organically grown groups.

To answer the question, I decided to just sit in a cafe and write what poured out of my head. So here you go; it reads like a mix of confessions, a novel and a magazine. When asked to contribute to this chapter my 'not good enough' story kicked in. . . . I can't write academic papers with references and intelligent prose; my strength is communicating with ordinary people in ordinary words that they understand, and not so much with intelligent therapists who see the world from a lens that's different to mine. Like Siobhan and Gavin, I also pushed it out of my head for a few weeks (with less reflection whilst out running) but finally recognised that as a clinician who feels my calling is to find the best way to communicate well with family members, and whoever else constitutes the system around a person with brain injury, I ought to practice what I preach and take a step out of my comfort zone.

To set a context, I should probably say a little about my family. I grew up in a stereotypically working-class family. My dad was a welder and my mum a hairdresser. They were kind and encouraging, their strong work ethic didn't allow days off school for anything other than terminal illness and my homecoming reward was always meat and two veg. My understanding of what a 'normal' family was comes from my own experience, plus our one week's break each year at a holiday camp and the soaps on television. We lived in a small village where everyone socialised in the local working men's club once a week, with very little diversity of culture or religion.

I worked very hard at school, but my parents didn't know what subjects I was taking or that an E didn't actually stand for Excellent. I dropped out of college and went to work in the local supermarket. A year later I was bored, and when my boyfriend refused to marry me, I followed up a suggestion a customer made about trying my A levels again. Throughout my career I have been very much in touch with my own sense of feeling like an unintelligent misfit surrounded by eloquent colleagues. In training, placements were easier as I was able to work with clients who came from families like mine. I realised I got on better with my customers than with my colleagues. I felt guilty about that; after all we were supposed to have clear boundaries. I had been told to keep people from seeing that we were also flawed human beings trying to find our own path. As time went on I began to specialise in brain injury, eventually earning the title of consultant clinical neuropsychologist specialising in neurorehabilitation. I saw that usually the person with the brain injury has a significant, but often small, part to play in the rehabilitation process.

It was a bit like a TV drama, where everyone around the injured person wasn't necessarily following the same script. I recall a conversation with my then-NHS manager 15 years ago about not spending too much time talking to people other than the 'referred person'. My puzzle was how do you work with a catastrophically injured person with physical, cognitive and emotional deficits when they were perfectly content and seemed oblivious to the impact of their injuries on themselves or others around them?

When there is a major incident on hospital TV dramas, the medics first attend to those who are experiencing the highest levels of physical distress. When I complete an initial assessment for someone who has sustained a brain injury, I often still feel that I have arrived at the site of a major incident, but the people who are in greatest distress are frequently not the injured person but their parents, their grandparents, their children, even the local GP, church pastor and friend. I wasn't far into my work with people with brain injury before I started attending to these people first. I recognised that the injured person would have no hope of recovery if all the people around them were so physically or mentally ill that they were psychologically unavailable to help. The bible describes a healthy church as a human body; some body parts are really small, but if they are not functioning well, the body as a whole can't thrive. Our role as neuropsychologists is to assess which body parts are bleeding most heavily and the impact that is having on other parts of the system, but we must also spot the healthy organs who can provide temporary or permanent support to get the body system working to its maximum potential.

For the first time, I realised I knew the language of ordinary people, and that was a strength when working within brain injury. Of course, not everybody with a brain injury is from a working-class background, but there is a skew in this direction potentially due to risk taking, education, coping skills and occupational choices. I knew about the social club and the soaps and could use analogies that were familiar. Irrespective of background though, many families find themselves in a new world of litigation and healthcare systems, and they benefit from jargon-free explanations. As the lead neuropsychologist in my local NHS department, I was able to include family members within my referral criteria. I worked harder to understand what life had been like for everyone before the uninvited guest of brain injury smashed its way into their lives.

I facilitated my first relatives' group 12 years ago. Twenty people came and the room was buzzing as people realised they were not alone. I later found out this is called the Principal of Universality. This group was self-sustaining for nine years. Since that first group formed, I advocated for groups in many different shapes and sizes, usually organically grown: for relatives, support workers, health professionals and most recently children. I always start with a one-off meeting and see what happens. I think I am right in remembering that Kreutzer, Marwitz, Hsu, Williams, and Riddick (2007) suggested if you have limited resources, female relatives might be a priority because they are vulnerable to developing clinical symptoms of anxiety and distress. Perhaps that's why a group that currently seems to be thriving is a female relatives' group. I introduced three of the women who I noticed were similar in age and background, and six more have since emerged. We meet quarterly, with dates coordinated on a what's app group. Each time I introduce a simple life enhancing idea like practising gratitude, thought management or keeping a journal, but most of the two hours is spent by informal discussion, information sharing and group problem solving. I wonder if building sustainable community support models is 'legitimate' systemic work?

In 2008, I was trying to provide as many interventions as possible to families within the NHS. A common fear for families that kept coming up was how children are impacted when a parent has a brain injury. These fears were a recurrent theme for adults I assessed with long-term conditions like MS, Parkinson's, Huntington's or stroke. I struggled to find attractive written information to share with younger children but also teenagers. I found a few older publications but felt the intended message was overly negative. I wanted something to explain the facts about cognitive and emotional and behavioural symptoms but also to acknowledge that young adults might experience difficult thoughts and feelings and to suggest age appropriate ways they could best manage how they felt without turning to negative coping strategies. I asked all the families I had worked with about whether their young people might want to help me produce the resource I wanted. Ten young people aged 9–19 volunteered, and over the next six years we produced seven publications to reassure young people that everything they were thinking and feeling was normal, and that most children thrive post parental brain injury and may even be more resilient than other children their age. This group of young people was the catalyst for an ongoing group called CAN – children and neurology. We meet three times a year to have fun and learn a little about minds and brains but mostly to enjoy time with others in the same situation.

I am not a pure 'systemicist' . . . most recently I have become inspired by the ACT (Acceptance and Commitment Therapy, Hayes, 2004); one of the things I like about this approach is its emphasis on the fact that we as professionals are as flawed as the people we seek to help, and that people are stuck rather than broken.

I am stuck now in my writing.

To summarise, I suppose I would like to say that we all have different genetics and backgrounds that we bring to the system of clinical neuropsychology and to the injured systems we encounter around our clients. This difference, of course, tints the lenses that we use to peer out at the world. For this reason, we cannot easily disentangle our own relationship experiences from our clinical work, and systemic practice teaches us to acknowledge this and to use this as a resource – a strength, if you like. For me, this meant I took the richness of my family and community experiences to help others rebuild their communities; this is the biggest source of long-term support available. I formulate reflectively. I bounce ideas around in my head and in group supervisions, comparing the client presentation with my own experience of being in the room with them, against my own 'norms' for families and of course wonder about whether this is 'right' and what I 'ought to be doing', comparing it with publications I read. I too use a mishmash of models, but the way in which I use them, and focus on family support, has been recognised by others as systemic (with the small 's' that Siobhan talks about). Can our work be 'systemic' if we don't use two-way mirrors, reflecting teams or long words? I do a lot of reflection on my own practice and try to put a mirror to us as professionals to avoid getting stuck in constricting positions that limit our flexibility and creativity. I am constantly looking for new ways to support family members affected by brain injury, not just partners or parents or couples but also children, siblings, and thinking generally about the meaning of the injury to the socially constructed identity of the injured person when their role in their family changes so radically. My own family was rooted in loyalty, patience, community and the ordinariness of life, and it is this ordinariness that paradoxically (probably) makes my contribution to neuropsychology unique.

Barry: an illustrative case study, presented by Richard

In my work in neurorehabilitation, I once worked with a consultant who found the messiness of families overwhelming and pretended he couldn't see them. Like a pre-operational child, for as long as he kept his eyes shut he could convince himself that nothing else existed, screening out the background interpersonal noise whilst performing his pharmacological alchemy. Whilst it is one way of dealing with the messiness, eventually you do have to open your eyes.

Barry suffered a catastrophic brain injury aged 34, although his sister's response to its horribleness was not what his Case Manager was accustomed to. They had spent over two decades supervising, supporting and sharing the responsibility associated with their younger brother's drug dependency problems. They had become desensitised to sitting on plastic chairs in disinfected hospital waiting areas drinking lukewarm liquid out of polystyrene cups waiting for the duty doctor. Barry's injury was yet another chapter in the family story of anxiety, crisis management and collective problem solving, perpetually seeking to minimise the impact of his self-destructive behaviours. Discharged to his own home with daytime support, I became actively involved after Barry stole drugs from an unlocked cupboard during a supervised hospital visit to see his father, recently diagnosed with dementia, in the local hospital.

There was an air of desperation in the case manager's voice when she called me. The task of seeking to reassure, repair and rebuild relationships between Barry's sisters and the support team seemed to be failing; his sisters described inescapable feelings of being unable to trust the team with the challenging task of supporting their brother. Suddenly, we found ourselves part of the family kaleidoscope, bridging the gaps that had been created between Barry, the support team and his sisters, trying to understand and explain the new pattern.

For me, working systemically is as much a part of neurorehabilitation as 3T MRI scans, baclofen pumps and communication aids. Over 20 years of looking in on the kaleidoscopes means that some of the patterns seem reassuringly familiar like the structural similarity of an MRI brain scan. However, like the scan image, closer inspection reveals its unique order and disorder.

Ostensibly, the backcloth to Barry's brain injury wasn't extraordinary. Unfortunately, personal histories of substance misuse and brain injury are common. However, the context of these events was as unique as the myriad permutations of neuronal and axonal changes following his brain trauma. My discussions with Barry's sisters highlighted our need to study this particular kaleidoscope more closely. The extent of the guilt associated with their decision to relinquish their role as Barry's main support seemed intolerable; the overwhelming and cumulative stress of their father's dementia diagnosis and Barry's injury had forced them to grudgingly accept their own fallibility. The task became one of renegotiating their role in Barry's care in a way that enabled them to manage the competing demands of their parent, sibling and own families. We resolved that their knowledge of Barry was incalculable, and the case manager also came to accept that they were the experts in dealing with their brother. They always had been.

I've never completed family therapy training and often find the therapeutic vernacular and techniques clunky, impersonal and insincere (although my formulations are invariably sprinkled with systemic ideas, and I am partial to a strategically placed circular question). The tweedy, beardy men and achingly cool 'third wave' CBT zealots might derive some comfort from the illusory certainty that their intrapsychic, straw men arguments afford them. However, I prefer the safe uncertainty that systemic work brings to my work with people after brain injury, whilst always endeavouring to keep my eyes wide open.

Reflections

We make no apology for the chatty and folksy style of this chapter – maybe a little too wordy for our benevolent editor but very true to our ethos and ourselves. This chapter has had a slow and long gestation. It has brewed and matured in the vat of time but surely benefitted by the added pinches of separate and reflected voices. As we've intimated all along, birthing a chapter in systemic work has been no different than the clinical work we write about. We hope we've made you think, to both feel emboldened by what you do and challenged to take things further.

Systemic and family therapies can be obscured by, and hide-bound by, impenetrable language, the need for teams and personnel and a sometimes confusing epistemology. We would and could defend the place of all these things – the language is a seed bed of thought and creativity, the teams the very agar gel to grow the discipline. However, hey ho, that's not what the average clinician, whether in an NHS or private healthcare environment, actually sees or needs. We sincerely hope that the reader feels emboldened to try out and practice, but do get supervision! It's the systemic mindset that's the most important thing, all in all. Accept the team bells and whistles if you can get them, but apply your mindset if that's all you've got.

References

Betteridge, S., Cotterill, E., & Murphy, P. (2017). Rehabilitation of challenging behaviour in community settings: The Empowerment Behavioural Management Approach (EMBA). In B. Wilson, G. Winegardener, C. M. Van Heugten, & T. Onsworth (Eds.), *Neuropsychological rehabilitation: An international handbook*. Oxon: Routledge.

Borrell-Carrió, F., Suchman, A. L., & Epstein, R. M. (2004). The biopsychosocial model 25 years later: Principles, practice, and scientific inquiry. *Annals of Family Medicine*, 2(6), 576–582.

Bowen, C., Hall, T., Newby, G., Walsh, B., Weatherhead, S., & Yeates, G. (2009). The impact of brain injury on relationships across the lifespan and across school, family and work contexts. *Human Systems: The Journal of Therapy, Consultation & Training*, 20(1), 65–80.

Bowen, C., Yeates, G., & Palmer, S. (2010). *A relational approach to rehabilitation: Thinking about relationships after brain injury*. London: Karnac Books.

Burnham, J. (2013). Developments in social GGRRAAACCEEESSS: Visible–invisible, voiced-unvoiced. In I. Krause (Ed.), *Culture and reflexivity in systemic psychotherapy: Mutual perspectives*. London: Karnac Books.

Carr, A. (2012). *Family therapy: Concepts, process and practice*. Hoboken, NJ: Wiley-Blackwell.

Cronen, V. E., Pearce, W. B., & Harris, L. M. (1982). The coordinated management of meaning: A theory of communication. In F. E. X. Dance (Ed.), *Human communication theory: Comparative essays* (pp. 61–89). New York: Harper & Row.

Engel, G. (1980). The clinical application of the biopsychosocial model. *American Journal of Psychiatry, 137,* 535–544.

Hawton, K., Salkovskis, P., Kirk, J., & Clark, D. (1994). *Cognitive behaviour therapy for psychiatric problems.* Oxford: Oxford Medical Publications.

Hayes, S. C. (2004). Acceptance and commitment therapy, relational frame theory, and the third wave of behavior therapy. *Behavior Therapy, 35,* 639–665.

Hoffman, L. (1993). *Exchanging voices: A collaborative approach to family therapy.* London: Karnac Books.

Howard, S. (2011). *Psychodynamic counselling in a nutshell* (3rd ed.). Los Angeles, CA: Sage Publications.

James Nathan Miller Quotes. (n.d.). *BrainyQuote.com.* Retrieved February 19, 2018, from www.brainyquote.com/quotes/james_nathan_miller_172017

James Nathan Miller Quotes. (n.d.). *BrainyQuote.com.* Retrieved July 10, 2018, from www.brainyquote.com/quotes/james_nathan_miller_172017

Johnson, S. M., & Greenberg, L. S. (1987). Emotionally focused marital therapy: An overview. *Psychotherapy: Theory, Research, Practice, Training, 24*(3S): 552–560.

Jones, V., & Reeve, D. (2014). *DISsing the social GGRRAAACCEEESSS.* Paper presented at AFT Annual Conference: IRREVERENCE – (Dis)respect, Freedoms, Loyalty, Ethics & Survival, Adelphi Hotel, Liverpool, 18–20 September.

Judd, D., & Wilson, S. L. (2005). Psychotherapy with brain injury survivors: An investigation of the challenges encountered by clinicians and their modifications to therapeutic practice. *Brain Injury, 19,* 437–449.

Kabat-Zinn, J. (1990). *Full Catastrophe Living:* Using the wisdom of your body and mind to face stress, pain and illness. New York: Random House Inc.

Klonoff, P. S., Lamb, D. G., & Henderson, S. W. (2001). Outcomes from milieu-based neurorehabilitation at up to 11 years post-discharge. *Brain Injury, 15*(5), 413–428.

Kreutzer, J., Marwitz, J., Hsu, N., Williams, K., & Riddick, A. (2007). Marital stability after brain injury: An investigation and analysis. *Neurorehabilitation, 22,* 53–59.

Lakoff, G., & Johnson, M. (1980). Conceptual metaphor in everyday language. *The Journal of Philosophy, 77*(8), 453–486.

Levine, B., Schweizer, T., O'Connor, C., Turner, G., Gillingham, S., Stuss, D. T. . . . Robertson, I. H. (2011). Rehabilitation of executive functioning in patients with frontal lobe brain damage with goal management training. *Frontiers in Human Neuroscience, 5*(9), 1–9.

Malan, D. (1995). *Individual psychotherapy and the science of psychodynamics* (2nd ed.). Hoboken, NJ: CRC Press.

Mason, B. (1993). Towards positions of safe uncertainty. *Human Systems: Journal of Therapy, Consultation and Training, 4*(3–4).

McWilliams, N. (2004). *Psychoanalytic psychotherapy: A practitioner's guide.* New York: Guilford Press.

Newby, G. J., Bushell, S., Cotter, I., & Nangle, N. (2004). Therapist "hear thyself": Using e-mail and debrief to acknowledged therapists' stories in narrative group work. *Clinical Psychology, 37,* 27–34.

Newby, G. J., & Coetzer, R. (2012). Facing down the elephant in the room: Making your CPD Log a successful part of your practice and development. *Clinical Psychology Forum, 236,* 46–49.

Newby, G. J., & Coutzer, R. (2013a). The use of emails and texts in psychological therapy after acquired brain injury. In G. Newby, R. Coetzer, A. Daisley, & S. Weatherhead (Eds.), *Practical neuropsychological rehabilitation in acquired brain injury: A guide for working clinicians.* London: Karnac Books.

Newby, G. J., & Coetzer, R. (2013b). Information technology: Augmenting psychological therapy and a new dimension in working with clients. *Neuro-disability & Psychotherapy, 1*, 213–228.

Newby, G. J., & Thorn, T. (2003). Working systemically with older adults in a multidisciplinary team: A journey from family therapy to systemic practice. *PSIGE Newsletter, 83*, 27–32.

Newby, G. J., & Weatherhead, S. (2013). Thinking creatively about CPD. In G. Newby, R. Coetzer, A. Daisley, & S. Weatherhead (Eds.), *Practical neuropsychological rehabilitation in acquired brain injury: A guide for working clinicians.* London: Karnac Books.

Orlinsky, D. E., & Howard, K. I. (1986). Process and outcome in psychotherapy. In S. L. Garfield & A. E. Berglov (Eds.), *Handbook of psychotherapy and behaviour change* (3rd ed., pp. 311–383). New York: Wiley-Blackwell.

Orlinksy, D. E., & Howard, K. I. (1995). Unity and diversity among psychotherapies: A comparative perspective. In B. Bongar & L. E. Beutler (Eds.), *Comprehensive textbook of psychotherapy* (pp. 3–23). Oxford: Oxford University Press.

Palmer, S., & Herbert, C. (2016). Friendships and intimacy: Promoting the maintenance and development of relationships in residential neurorehabilitation. *NeuroRehabilitation, 38*(3), 291–298.

Pearce, W. B., & Cronen, V. (1980). *Communication, action, and meaning: The creation of social realities.* New York: Praeger.

Pilgrim, D., & Treacher, A. (1992). *Clinical psychology observed.* London: Routledge.

Prigatano, G. P. (1999). *Principles of neuropsychological rehabilitation.* New York: Oxford University Press.

Rockland, L. (1989). *Supportive therapy: A psychodynamic approach.* New York: Basic Books.

Selvini, M. P., Boscolo, L., Cecchin, G., & Prata, G. (1980). Hypothesizing – Circularity – Neutrality: Three guidelines for the conductor of the session. *Family Process, 19*, 3–12.

Thomsen, I. V. (1992). Late psychosocial outcome in severe traumatic brain injury. Preliminary results of a third follow-up study after 20 years. *Scandinavian Journal of Rehabilitation Medicine, Supplement, 26*, 142–152.

Vetere, A., & Dallos, R. (2003). *Working systemically with families: Formulation, intervention and evaluation.* London: Karnac Books.

Weatherhead, S. J., Coetzer, R., Daisley, A., Newby, G., Yeates, G., & Calvert, P. (2013). Therapy and engagement. In G. Newby, R. Coetzer, A. Daisley, & S. Weatherhead (Eds.), *Practical neuropsychological rehabilitation in acquired brain injury: A guide for working clinicians.* London: Karnac Books.

Weatherhead, S. J., & Newby, G. J. (2011). *Warehouse of responsibilities: A group for survivors of a brain injury.* Retrieved from www.theinstituteofnarrativetherapy.com/Papers/Warehouse%20of%responsibility.doc

Wood, R. L., & Alderman, N. (2011). Applications of operant learning theory to the management of challenging behavior after traumatic brain injury. *The Journal of Head Trauma Rehabilitation, 26*, 202–211.

Wood, R. L., Liossi, C., & Wood, L. (2005). The impact of head injury neurobehavioural sequelae on personal relationships: Preliminary findings. *Brain Injury, 19*(10), 845–851.

9

MIND-BODY INTERVENTIONS IN NEUROREHABILITATION

Giles N. Yeates

Overview

Traditional psychological approaches to neurorehabilitation in the West rely on seated-based talking therapies that make inevitable demands of a survivor's ability to control their mental and physical experience. In contrast, mind-body approaches from Eastern Asia have evolved over thousands of years to offer a range of different positions and relationships between an individual and their mental experience. The body is often a key resource in defining a unique relationship with mind, and as such may offer novel therapeutic opportunities for people with neuro–disability. This chapter will cover the two prominent mind-body traditions used with acquired brain injury survivors, Yoga and Tai Ji. The reader is encouraged to read this chapter alongside the mindfulness chapter (Chapter 3) by Niels Detert.

Introduction

Psychological needs following Acquired Brain Injury (ABI) are often prominent, including anxiety, depression, anger and irritability, post-traumatic stress and struggles to adjust to the condition (Williams & Evans, 2003). These often occur alongside physical restrictions (reduced, mobility, balance, sensation), cognitive impairments and strain in interpersonal relationships, with progressive social isolation developing over time (Elsass & Kinsella, 1987). A closer examination of survivor's experience of psychological distress post–injury highlights core existential threats to identity and selfhood. Goldstein (1959) was the first to describe a catastrophic reaction in survivors with left anterior brain lesions, and Luria (1975) wrote about the 'shattered world' of a survivor of parietal damage. Themes of fragmentation of self are common in survivors' accounts (such as in Nochi's work on identity in stroke survivors, Nochi, 1997, 1998a, 1998b, 2000).

Others describe a sense of alienation from pre-injury self and inertia, feeling like a shell of a person (Sacks, 1973; Yeates, 2015). These aspects of self-disturbance are complex and nuanced and difficult to alleviate through traditional forms of emotional support. These existential crises also trigger crises of faith for those with relevant belief systems. Psychological difficulties can also be intertwined with physical and cognitive impairments, such as an intensification of distress during states of neurological fatigue and difficulties managing negative thoughts/experiences in mind as a result of working memory/attention deficits.

The complexity and interconnected, multidomain nature of post-injury difficulties require innovative options of support that address body, mind (with all of its unique forms of disturbance in ABI) and social relationships. However, forms of support commonly offered in ABI services are often demarcated and punctuated by professional boundaries and are time-limited. As a result, physiotherapy interventions can be compromised by the impact of cognitive difficulties (e.g., initiation and/or memory) and emotional influences (low mood, anxiety). Survivors themselves often prioritise a need for continued physiotherapy beyond the time-limits of public service provision rather than seek psychological support, despite others around them identifying survivor adjustment needs.

Traditional paradigms of psychological therapy dominate ABI services' provision of emotional support for survivors, as evident in this book, and are supported by adjunctive cognitive rehabilitation strategies and technological adaptations (Yeates, 2014) to mitigate the potentially negative impact of cognitive difficulties on therapy outcome (e.g., Yeates et al., 2008). However, all of these are based on the traditional, seated, talking-therapy format. A ubiquitous seated verbal exchange for an hour is not a sufficiently flexible and innovative response to the myriad of survivors' altered relationships with their minds post-injury. Cognitive difficulties such as working memory, attentional and executive impairments can result in a restricted ability to manage the content of one's mind, even to access positive/alternative thoughts, and exceptions to adversarial life events, as required by many therapy orientations. Attentional/arousal difficulties may mean it is hard for a survivor to focus on a set of ideas whilst sitting down in conversation for an hour (as would barriers to seating arising from physical disability), and communication difficulties such as aphasia may preclude a conversational-based form of emotional support altogether.

A direct engagement with dimensions of spirituality and existential meaning are commonly omitted from psychology sessions (and those of other rehabilitation professionals). Finally, the social isolation that characterises survivors' longer-term trajectories is insufficiently addressed by time-limited psychosocial intervention, mirrored by a range of barriers to survivors' satisfactory access to community leisure and social resources for the general population. This is despite the demonstration of the value of multiple, long-term social group membership for survivor post-injury identity (Haslam et al., 2008).

To conclude, a mind-body community psychosocial intervention for survivors in ABI, that is long-term in remit, available in the community and has the potential to support deeper dimensions of spirituality and meaning, remains outstanding. Clinicians working with neurological patients across different service contexts have looked beyond talking therapy paradigms to find novel and flexible approaches to emotional and existential support that may adequately respond to the aforementioned diversity and complexity. To this end, Eastern spiritual, philosophical and health cultivation practices have become increasingly accessed as a resource.

Eastern mind-body practices in neurorehabilitation

Asian spiritual traditions are both ancient and diverse, operationalising different ideas of the mind and spirit. One common thread running through the three traditions that have influenced published neurorehabilitation work to date, Buddhism, Vedic traditions and Daosim, is a focus on using the body to manage the mind and create opportunities for psychological and spiritual growth. As such, the approach to mind and the specific mind-body practices from each offer new opportunities to survivors of acquired brain injury in managing emotional and existential challenges (Yeates, 2015; Yeates & Farrell, 2014, 2018).

Mindfulness approaches in neurorehabilitation are covered elsewhere in this book (Detert, Chapter 3). In an attempt to widen the accessibility of mindfulness practices to those who would struggle solely with seated mediation (the main vehicle of mindfulness practice in the majority of clinical interventions), some clinicians have used martial arts movements to create new interventions for those with complex needs, and have considered the value of such for people with neurological conditions (Russell, 2011; Russell & Tatton-Ramos, 2014). This chapter will consider two mind-body traditions, yoga and Tai Ji (Tai Chi), that centrally use the body and breath as meditational foci when working with people with complex physical health needs, including for the purposes of this book, stroke, traumatic brain injury and other forms of ABI.

Yoga

There is a considerable appeal of approaches that involve the body more centrally in meditative practice, and so offer additional clinical gains such as increased balance, postural control, mobility, strength and flexibility, and so it can simultaneously contribute to both physical and psychological goals post-injury. Yoga means 'yoke' or 'union', a system of different meditative and lifestyle practices from the Indian subcontinent that is intertwined with the Vedic tradition and Hinduism. One of eight stands of yoga that is most commonly associated with the name is the practice of *asana* or adopting physical poses (that work the practitioner's flexibility, balance and strength), whilst simultaneously regulating the breath and focusing the mind.

The application of Yoga in a neurorehabilitation setting has been described in several reviews and individual studies of stroke survivors (Bastille & Gill-Body, 2004; Lazaridou, Philbrook, & Tzika, 2013; Lynton, Kligler, & Shiflett, 2007), reporting gains in physical and cognitive functioning alongside reduction in stress. Yogic movements have traditionally been included in mindfulness-based stress reduction protocols with neurological patients, such as in a stroke study by Moustgaard, Bedard, and Felteau (2007). Donnelly, Linnea, Grant, and Lichtenstein (2014) demonstrated the feasibility of a yoga intervention for survivors of traumatic brain injury, reporting indications of benefits in aspects of quality of life relative to a control group. Yeates and colleagues (2014) demonstrated gains in the reduction of anxiety and fatigue across survivors in their single-case analysis of a pilot yoga group within a community brain injury service, and gains in respiratory, physical and psychological functioning have been reported in a pilot by Silverthorne, Khalsa, Gueth, DeAvilla, and Pansini (2012). Detailed brain injury case study accounts have been provided by Shravat (2014) and Schmidt, Miller, Van Puymbroeck, and Schalk (2016). Participants with epilepsy were found to benefit from yoga plus acceptance and commitment therapy (Lundgren, Dahl, Yardi, & Melin, 2008) and a yoga/ meditation protocol (Rajesh, Jayachandran, Mohandas, & Radhakrishnan, 2006), with gains including reduced seizure frequency and increased quality of life.

Following the suggestions by Russell (2011) that the body can be more centrally incorporated into meditative practice to widen the accessibility of such practices to service users who struggle with attention, these yoga interventions within neurorehabilitation offer both new paradigms for emotional support and concurrent physical gains too. In relation to spiritual care, the aforementioned survivor experience of fragmentation may be uniquely approached by the aim in yogic asana practice of unifying mind, body and spirit in an embodied meditative tradition.

Tai Ji (Tai Chi)

There is one further mind-body tradition from Asia that has been repeatedly demonstrated to offer concurrent psychological and physical gains for neurological populations: Tai Ji (TJ, often written erroneously as Tai Chi), developed in China during the 12th/13th century CE, is often credited as the creation of Daoist (Taoist) priests, which was later spread to the wider Jinese populace and pioneered through unique styles linked to particular families (Yeates, 2015). TJ practice is characterised by slow, soft flowing movements of all parts of the body, alongside breath regulation and deep psychological immersion in the movements. It is practiced as both a martial art (and is indeed the world's most popular martial art) and health cultivation practice. TJ will form the main focus of this chapter going forward, but here I will introduce the main findings from the rapidly growing clinical evidence base of the use of TJ with different neurological populations. In the subsequent sections of this chapter, I will explore the theological and psychological dimension of TJ practice and how this may inform future use of TJ within neurorehabilitation.

The scientific study of TJ in the general population has demonstrated gains in physical, cognitive and emotional functioning plus biophysical structural differences for regular practitioners (Jahnke et al., 2012). A review of TJ group trials with long-term complex conditions concluded there was evidence of both physical and psychological gains of TJ practice within these groups (Zhang et al., 2012). The strongest and most established evidence base for the use of TJ with ABI is with stroke – primarily evidence of gains in physical functioning from participation in TJ groups.

With regard to reviews of the stroke rehabilitation literature, Lyu and colleagues (2018) found TJ to have an overall beneficial effect on activities of daily living, balance, limb motor function, walking quality, mood and sleep from low quality evidence-based studies. Qin, Wei, Liu, and Zhu (2016) found that when compared with standard physically orientated rehabilitation, TJ conferred significant gains in the areas of balance function, gait speed, anxiety and quality of life, in their meta-analysis of 15 eligible studies from both the English and Chinese language scientific literature. In contrast no advantages were evident for survivor levels of depression or functional walking quality. Ding (2012) concluded from a review of five studies that TJ confers advantageous gains to stroke survivors in the domains of balance, mobility, quality of life, anxiety and depression. Gains in balance are the most replicated outcome across studies, concluded in reviews by Wu and colleagues (2018), Yan Li, Wang, Liu, and Zhang (2018) and Zou, Wang, Chen, and Wang (2018). A systematic review and meta-analysis across multiple neurological conditions by Winser, Kannan, Pang, Smith, and Tsang (2018) concluded that there is strong evidence for improvement in balance and reduction in falls in people with either Parkinson's Disease or stroke, with weaker evidence for this outcome in other conditions. Similar practices, such as baduanjin qi gong, have also been shown across studies to improve balance and other aspects of physical functioning, whilst reducing levels of depression, amongst other indices (Zou, Yeung et al., 2018).

In terms of specific studies, a large sample (n = 244) study by Xie and colleagues (2018) identified gains in motor functioning, fear of falling and depression when compared with a balance training control intervention. Taylor-Piliae et al. (2014) found Yang style TJ for older stroke survivors (> 50) group to have had fewer falls than aerobic and treatment as usual control groups. Both TJ and aerobic control better aerobic endurance than treatment as usual. No group effect was found for perceived mental health – all groups reported this. Wang and colleagues (2010) found a positive differences for a TJ stroke group on measures of sleep quality/daytime dysfunction (including fatigue) and depressive symptoms. TJ interventions have been shown to improve standing balance in an older adults sample (Au-Yeung, Hui-Chan, & Tang, 2009), and a sample of community-based stroke survivors reported gains in both general functioning and mood, alongside no adverse effects for practitioners (Hart et al., 2004). Hwang and colleagues (2019) found that an adapted TJ group for stroke survivors with hemiplegia that last for one year (ten participants completed all sessions) was characterised by improvements in balance, self-efficacy and flexibility on quantitative measures, alongside identification within qualitative interviews highlighting positive improvements for participants in physical and psychological functioning, social support and activities of daily living. In a case study of a stroke survivor with expressive aphasia, Yeates (in press) reported clinically significant and reliable gains on measures of depression and fatigue-related psychosocial functioning, plus detailed qualitative data following the survivor's attendance at a six-month TJ group. A qualitative analysis of stroke survivor experiences in a TJ group by Desrochers, Kairy, Pan, Corriveau, and Tousignant (2016) highlighted simultaneous perceived physical and psychological benefits by participants. Interestingly, TJ has been applied to intentionally reduce risk factors to prevent the incidence of stroke for those who are at risk (Chan, Sit, & Chair, 2017).

Another key subgroup of acquired brain injury, traumatic brain injury (TBI) has been investigated in TJ studies, but using much smaller samples. Gemmell and Leathem (2006) have studied the psychosocial benefits for nine TBI survivors from a brief (six weeks) TJ group intervention, and reported participants' improved levels of sadness, confusion, anger, tension, fear and increased energy on visual analogue scales. Blake and Batson (2006) used a randomised design to demonstrate improvements in mood and self-esteem but not physical functioning in a TJ versus control group (20 participants in each condition). The authors concluded that their results were inconclusive as a recommendation for the use of TJ with TBI survivors. Finally, Shapira, Chelouche, Yanai, Kaner, and Szold (2001) report three case studies where TBI survivors who had participated in TJ reported gains in mobility and feelings of security whilst walking.

Gains from TJ have also been reported for people with cerebellar ataxia (balance and functional independence, Winser, Kannan, Pang, & Tsang, 2017; Winser et al., 2018). Quinn and Jones (2012) reported a range of psychosocial gains following completion of a TJ group for people with a variety of neurological conditions. Yeates and colleagues (submitted; Yeates, 2019, in press) also report positive single case outcomes for a small group of survivors of ABI following a six-month TJ group but also draw attention to significant diversity in this group and the influence of such on the range of outcomes within the group

In summary, the existing literature points reliably to a range of physical functioning gains across neurological conditions, although the evidence is strongest and most reliable in stroke. Conclusions for other conditions are limited by small sample sizes and differing outcome measures. There are two key problems with this literature as a whole, however. A general critique is that the most rigorously designed studies have optimised participant homogeneity by excluding those participants with significant cognitive difficulties alongside their physical impairments (e.g., Taylor-Piliae et al., 2014). This then creates a barrier to applying the findings of these studies to the users of services described earlier in this chapter, who are struggling with multiple domains of disability (Yeates, 2015, 2018, 2019, in press; Yeates et al., submitted). More recently, Hwang and colleagues (2019) have been the first to describe physical adaptations to a TJ group for stroke survivors with hemiplegia.

Furthermore, most studies have operationalised physical functioning measures as the primary outcome only. Where psychological functioning has been additionally studied, it is clear from the findings in this section that frequent gains in anxiety and depression are found by investigators. However these have not been the main focus of each study, nor have investigators offered explanatory frameworks to explain the link between performing TJ movements and emotional wellbeing. Burschka, Keune, Oy, Oschman, and Kuhn (2014) did offer mindfulness as a possible explanatory framework for these empirical associations, but as we'll explore later, this is not the key mind-body framework that TJ experts use to guide their practice.

Daoist frameworks for Tai Ji, Qi Gong and flow-based practices

The omissions in the scientific literature described previously are all the more significant when one considers that those expert TJ practitioners who practice the most, for the longest and prioritise this practice above other aspects of life all hold the internal, subjective (psychological) dimension to be central to their practice. Taijiquan, means the representation of the universe (in the Daoist view) through bodily movement. It is still practiced by the Daoist monastic community to this day, as well as millions of other practitioners worldwide, of all ages, backgrounds and abilities. For the Daoist monk TJ masters, despite their mastery and prowess of physical movements, balance and coordination, their focus is on their internal experience in harmony with both their bodily movements and wider universal natural processes, all connected within their view of natural laws and organisation. This is a unique bio-psycho-social-spiritual-ecological framework, which will be explored here.

Daoism is a key indigenous religion of China. Practiced by at least 20 million people in China and worldwide, Daoism was formalised in 2nd century CE but is thought to have developed from preceding shamanic beliefs and codeveloped in reciprocal dialogue with Chan Buddhism and Confucionism, the other two main spiritual-philosophical traditions in pre-communist China. The Daoist view of the divine is an emanating universal force that proceeds and evolves, underlying all the manifestations of change and transition in the natural world and wider universe. This process is called Dao, which translates as the 'way' or 'path'. Nature is a key source of inspiration to connect with the divine in Daoism, through the witnessing and harmonising of one's lifestyle with changing seasons, differing states and qualities of essential elements such as water (ice, fog, mist, rivers and lakes). This harmonisation of lifestyle is done via horticultural practices, herbology, musical and architectural styles and mind-body practices. The body is viewed as a manifestation of nature and subject to its laws (yin – receiving, embracing, yielding forces, and yang – emanating, protruding, opening forces). As such one's body, and the interrelationship between the body and the embodied mind is seen as a domain in which a Daoist can intentionally promote harmony with nature.

This harmonisation and health cultivation process in the level of body, mind and spirit is referred to as 'Neidan', or 'Inner Alchemy'. The practitioner aims to self-harmonise with natural processes and facilitate a key process of conversion – from their bodily essence/physical properties ('Jing') their physical attributes are used in service of breath regulation to stimulate and circulate a flow of vitality and life energy ('Qi') around the body. This circulation alters the mind and subjective experience of the practitioner, leading to expanded states of consciousness. These final processes are conceived as the domain of spirit ('Shen'), but different qualities of mind-spirit are anchored to specific mind-body physiological networks, with links to specific organs (including the heart, lungs, kidneys and liver). This echoes more contemporary developments in neuroscience that highlight interoceptive processes mediated by subcortical-viscera networks that are generative of consciousness (Damasio, 1999). This conversion of body-breath/life energy-spirit is completed by the highest converted essence being put back into the universe. As such the body, breath, mind and spirit are all vehicles and containers for a never-ending flow of universal change processes that permeate all things. The aim, then, is to minimise blocks and desynchronies that would obstruct this process.

The Neidan process is a core focus of seated Daoist meditational practices, but it is also the organiser for a range of mind-body practices such as TJ, qi gong (still or moving yogic practices that typically involve greater repetition of fewer movements than TJ) and gong fu (kung fu – faster and more dynamic practices with a clear martial focus). Furthermore, music, chanting of hymns and scriptures, horticulture, cooking and eating, architecture, divination and sleeping are also used as lifestyle vehicles for Neidan to aim towards a constant trend towards harmonisation with nature and the divine.

Flow psychology

Therefore, in contrast to TJ as a physical practice only, we have a rich range of Daoist concepts that both guide internal experience during bodily practice and situate them within a wider ecological and lifestyle context. One limitation is that these concepts are esoteric and not easily accessible. These core concepts do however overlap significantly with some key ideas within Western positive psychology, a broad contemporary influence on neurorehabilitation (Cullen et al., 2018; Evans, 2011; Evans & Cullen, in press, chapter x). Mihály Csíkszentmihályi (1990, 1997) has developed the concept of Flow, a concept which can potentially offer an explanatory bridge between Daoist terminology and scientific-clinical discourse (Yeates, 2015, 2018). Indeed, Csíkszentmihályi (1990) has explicitly identified another eastern mind-body tradition, yoga, as a purposefully designed flow activity:

> The similarities between Yoga and flow are extremely strong; in fact it makes sense to think that (Patanjali's system of) Yoga is a very thoroughly

planned Flow activity'; p 105, 'Therefore it is not unreasonable to view Yoga as one of the oldest and most systematic methods of producing the Flow experience.

(p. 105)

Csíkszentmihályi has primarily studied intense states of absorption in the domains of sport, music, creativity and work. Flow states are routinely described by practitioners as involving the dissolving of a self-state and loss of normal self-boundaries (loss of reflective self-consciousness), distortion of temporal experience, a merging of action and awareness where intention is not effortful, the activity concerned seeming to flow forth of its own accord. Practitioners feel intense wellbeing, ecstatic experiences at the time and part of something bigger than themselves. Importantly, those experiencing flow states in a particular activity have attained some level of mastery over that activity through practice and experience, such that there is a dimension of automaticity and diminution of effort. Practitioners across diverse fields consistently use a metaphorical language of creativity and action flowing forth, hence Csíkszentmihályi's term 'flow states'. Many of us know what it is to be 'in the flow', and the value of such, when we think about optimal times for our own performance and productivity. Flow has been associated with optimal psychological wellbeing (Csíkszentmihályi, 1990, 1997), and a specific focus on flow has been included in a positive psychotherapy intervention that was shown to be acceptable for survivors of acquired brain injury, with a recommendation for a future trial of this approach in ABI (Cullen et al., 2018).

Csíkszentmihályi acknowledged historical precursors to his psychological study of flow, notably religious thought from near and far Eastern traditions. Many faiths have historically articulated and practiced a desired goal to be at oneness with something greater, via dissolution of the boundaries of present sensory experience. In addition to Daoism these include: in Islam, Sufi Dervishes' practice of spinning and whirling. Furthermore in Vedic/Hindu thought a form of flow-like psychological absorption in an object of meditation, Samyama, is the goal in Raja Yoga and in fast forms of physical Yoga, flow states are explicitly the desired vehicle for self-transcendence. Finally, Gregorian chanting is a key flow practice in Christianity and the use of prayer beads and repetition of prayer forms/mantras in all the major faiths. The concept of flow is explicitly mentioned by exponents of the Daoist world-view, and famously by Bruce Lee:

Be like water . . . empty your mind, be formless, shapeless like water. If you put water in the cup, it becomes the cup. You put water in the bottle, it becomes the bottle. You put it in the teapot, it becomes the teapot. Now, water can flow or it can crash. Be water my friend.

(Little & Lee, 2000, TV Documentary)

We are always in a process of becoming and nothing is fixed. Have no rigid system in you, and you'll be flexible to change with the ever changing.

Open yourself and flow, my friend. Flow in the total openness of the living moment. If nothing within you stays rigid, outward things will disclose themselves. Moving, be like water. Still, be like a mirror. Respond like an echo.

(Lee, 2000, p. 13)

With change and transformation processes afforded such psychological and spiritual significance, the dimension of change is seen as the domain in which personal development occurs. This is commensurate with the focus across cultures and human experience on *liminality*, which has become an area of transdisciplinary academic and applied clinical interest. Liminal experiences are seen as self-experience within a phase of transition (between what someone once was and what they are becoming) and being of psychological value. Anthropologists have noted the centrality of liminal experience in rites of passage across cultures, where this phase (such as adolescent transition between childhood and adulthood) is marked by ceremony and symbolism. Narratives of passing through gates and portals permeate all of the major religions, be these processes of change in behaviour and learning or the unlocking of centres within the body. Psychotherapy too has been conceived as an arena where:

A new set of circumstances involve the dissolution of a former identity and the formation of a new identity. Between these two states, the condition of liminality suspends a person or system in what may appear to be an amorphous or ill-defined state.

(Elliot, 2011)

Growth and adaptation are viewed as emergent from such conditions. To link back to the experiences of ABI survivors, adjustment, awareness and post-injury growth can be limited by a rigid investment in pre-injury identity in a way that devalues post-injury change and closes down growth opportunities (Tyerman & Humphrey, 1984). A Daoist-focused exploration of the course of change itself rather than the privileging of one particular state in that journey may create new rehabilitation opportunities. An example would be comparing the relative attributes and limitations of different values and abilities at different points in time, in response to varying life conditions and demands post-injury

While there is clearly overlap between Daoist and positive psychological conceptualisation of flow states, the latter differs in emphasising explicit appraisal as a critical dimension. This includes assertions of flow components and conditions for flow, such as an individual's sense of personal control or agency, involvement in a task with a clear set of goals and progress and a task which provides immediate feedback and a simultaneous perception of high task challenges alongside high personal skill (Csikszentmihalyi, Abuhamdeh, & Nakamura, 2005; Shaffer, 2013). Whilst Daoist masters clearly have mastery of highly skilled practices such as martial arts, accounts of their subjective experiences during practice indicate a diminution of explicit appraisal processes generally and subjective absence of perceived challenge or personal skill (see 'The Taijiquan Classics', Davis, 2004). Furthermore, the psychological study of people in flow states has focused on those who have specific goals around performance (be this athletic or work productivity), with flow states being a dimension towards these outcomes. The Daoist TJ masters aspire specifically to enter into flow states and the opportunities for transcendence and wider harmony, irrespective of their performance (although it is clear that their physical and psychological abilities exceed most in the general population).

Using flow states to guide Tai Ji groups in neurorehabilitation

The extrapolation of concepts from Daoist psychology, by way of a translation with the Western concept of flow, has provided us with a new psychological tool to be used in clinical application. As there was once a time before people were using the mindfulness concept across a range of sectors, the concept of flow awaits a future explosion of clinical application. It is argued here (and in Yeates, 2015, 2018), that flow provides the core operationalisation of a psychological (and for some a spiritual) dimension in the formulation and implementation of TJ groups for people with neuro-disability. Flow is significant for TJ clinical interventions in two main ways: it (1) links the subjective experience of bodily movements with the evidenced psychological gains from TJ practice, and (2) builds on existing studies in positive psychology which identify a correlation between flow states and psychological wellbeing. This may offer a unique response to the existential disturbances to self-experience described earlier. To use the Daoist inspirations from the natural world, think of leaves floating in a stream. They are individual elements, but when moved simultaneously in the flow of currents and eddies in the stream, they are held in unison by a higher level of process or organisation. Similarly, the survivor of ABI, initially experiencing themselves as fragmented, 'in pieces', can be temporarily held together by the TJ movement sequence, which is also perhaps held together by moving in unison with fellow TJ practitioners (akin to a murmuration of starlings or a shoal of fish), and for some there may be an experience of synchrony and union with a higher principle – a transcendent experience.

Second, it can provide the specificity to optimise flow experience (with associated conditions of improved psychological wellbeing and the possibility of transcendence) for each practitioner in a bespoke fashion. If flow emerges from the optimal ratio of perceived challenge and ability to meet that challenge, then specific movements are chosen that fit this ration for each survivor (with their unique constellation of physical, cognitive, emotional and social needs). Furthermore, specific compensatory rehabilitation strategies are included as adjuncts to optimise the learning and practice of TJ (see Table 9.1, for examples), again to promote and optimise flow.

TABLE 9.1 Examples of adaptations to Tai Ji learning and practice for different post-stroke difficulties

Area of difficulty	Suggested adaptation
Mobility	Chair-based sequences and/or restricted standing TJ forms
Balance	Chair-based sequences, and/or TJ forms that have minimal weight and direction changes
Hemiplegia	Use of therapy bands, sticks and bilateral hand connection to mobilise mirroring upper-body movements, visual imagery of paralysed limb movement, focus on trunk movement to amplify functional movement of ipsilateral limbs
Fatigue	Do short sequences of instruction and movement, slowly increasing over time Regular breaks
Dyspraxia	Use tactile feedback and physical adjustments rather than relying on visual demonstration alone
Communication	Emphasis on visual and kinaesthetic teaching as opposed to verbal-based
Attention	Do short sequences of instruction and movement, slowly increasing over time Regular breaks
	Use of key phrases and words for optimal alerting qualities
Episodic memory/new learning	Focus on errorless learning (Wilson et al., 2010) in class to minimise the introduction of mistakes into the learning process
	For those that want to learn sequences at home, use of DVDs/internet videos to provide a guide between-session time and promote a greater number of repetition learning experiences
	Support the autonomous learning of a sequence through backward-chaining rather than traditional instruction
Topographical disorientation/ visuo-spatial difficulties in using allocentric or egocentric cues	Use grids marked on the floor to assist with changing directions of movement and posture shapes
Anxiety	Use of relaxing music, short teaching sequences
	Teach body-tension reduction and breath regulation strategies at the beginning of the class
	Reduce the learning/practice demands of the movements initially to increase confidence, then gently introducing progressively more challenging sequences
Low mood	Shorter learning/practice phases; pacing the progressive challenge of sequences as earlier, supporting achievements with praise and encouragement, emphasising the group fellowship and identity aspects of attendance
	Drawing comparison to embodied experience at the end of the session versus the beginning

The systematic use of flow in this way to optimise psychological wellbeing within TJ practice for survivors of ABI and people with other forms of disability would result in two different practitioners performing very different movement sequences (each with varying physical and psychological demands) and using very different compensatory strategies, but both enter into a similar state of flow within their practice (having arrived at it and entered into it through different routes). Within a TJ group intervention (a flow group, © Yeates, 2016), the session would be structured to offer both time devoted to individual learning of bespoke movements and also an additional segment of group movement sequences (accessible to all attendees) to facilitate the experience of group cohesion with others, plus a dedicated time for socialising and peer connection during a tea break.

This model of a TJ intervention for individuals or groups of ABI survivors is very different in scope and character from those protocols described in published studies. This is the author's current approach to TJ use as a clinical neuropsychologist, and the author awaits future controlled studies to confirm the core hypothesis – that optimising flow via the bespoke selection of TJ movements and use of compensatory strategies will result in more significant psychological gains for more practitioners than unadapted TJ groups. To provide more details on the value of TJ and the experience of flow for a survivor of ABI, a case study will be described in the next section.

Case example: Mark

Reported here is a case study from a six-month pilot TJ group (Yeates et al., submitted). Two very successful case study outcomes from this group are reported elsewhere (Yeates, 2019, in press), whereas here a modest set of outcomes for another participant is described to reflect those users of ABI community services that struggle with enduring and complex difficulties and the role of TJ within the lives of such people.

Mark is 44 and a survivor of at least two definitive neurological events. He developed a right acoustic neuroma, which grew aggressively and pushed down on surrounding structures, including the cerebellum and temporal lobe. This was surgically removed in 1999, but then Mark developed a CSF leak and later contracted meningitis on two subsequent occasions in the year post-surgery. Once medically stable he accessed support from a community neurorehabilitation service. He was actually referred from mental health services, who had been trying to treat longstanding anxiety, low mood and obsessive compulsive disorder for several years prior to Mark's diagnosis (he reports the presence of such difficulties since his early twenties) and one year post-surgery. Interventions included anti-depressant medication and cognitive-behavioural therapy for OCD, and both offered only partial relief from symptoms. The assessment phase of the community neurorehab team highlighted post-surgical/infection cognitive difficulties in speed of information processing, selective and sustained attention, working memory, goal-directed executive functions, cognitive flexibility and inhibitory control.

Physical challenges since the tumour resection have included problems with balance, headaches and momentary alterations to consciousness that are suspected to be complex partial seizures (responded to with anticonvulsant treatment). In addition neurological fatigue was an enduring problem and exacerbated low mood and anxiety (as did ruminative thought processes that had developed pre-morbidly but were exacerbated by the aforementioned attentional and executive difficulties). Mark constantly struggled with these ruminative patterns, which drained him and prevented him from realising his intentions to be productive as an artist.

When a six-month weekly pilot, a Tai Ji group was run at the service (Yeates et al., submitted), Mark was keen to take part. He completed 88% of the sessions (a significantly higher level of activity engagement than his participation in other community activities and rehabilitation sessions during the same period of time), learning how to regulate his breathing, move softly and use the movements as an embodied focus of attention, to progressively exit from periods of overthinking and high anxiety. As part of the research project, he completed questionnaires measuring anxiety and depression (Hospital Anxiety & Depression Scale, HADS, Zigmond & Snaith, 1983) and fatigue (Modified Fatigue Impact Scale, M-FIS, Fisk et al., 1994) on a repeating basis every week weeks. In addition, Mark completed a Quality of Life (Quality of Life after Brain Injury Inventory, QoLiBRI, ref) questionnaire prior to the first session and following the last session of the intervention. Clinical significance of changes in scores were determined using severity categories and cut-offs published for each scale, where the statistical reliability of score changes was evaluated using the Reliable Change Index (Jacobson & Truax, 1991).

Mark's scores on these measures before and after the six-month TJ group are reported in Table 9.2.

TABLE 9.2 Mark's mood, fatigue and quality of life data

Measure	Pre-TJ	Post-TJ	Significance?
HADS anxiety	17	14	Severe to moderate, not reliable
HADS depression	7	12	Borderline to moderate, reliable
MFIS total	51	39	Clinically significant and reliable
MFIS physical subscale	28	25	n/a
MFIS cognitive subscale	31	32	n/a
MFIS psychosocial	8	7	n/a
QoLiBRI total	80	79	No change

Source: HADS = Hospital Anxiety & Depression Scale; MFIS = Modified Fatigue Impact Scale; QoLIBRI = Quality of Life in Brain Injury Scale

Mark's scores on these measures across the four-week repeated measures data collection schedule graphed in Figures 9.1 and 9.2:

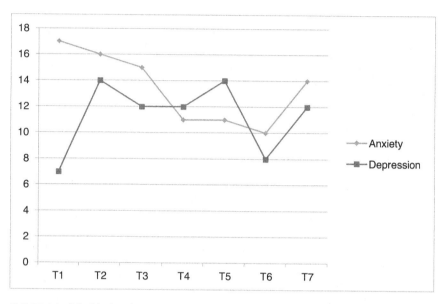

FIGURE 9.1 Mark's Anxiety & Depression (HADS) scores across sessions during the six-month Tai Ji group

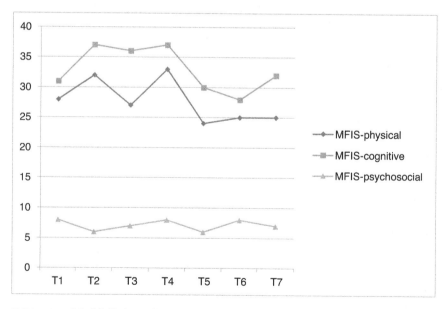

FIGURE 9.2 Mark's Fatigue (MFIS) scores across sessions during the six-month Tai Ji group

An examination of the scores highlight a mixed impact of the group on formal measures. Changes in Mark's anxiety were clinically significant (moving from the severe to moderate range on the HADS, with an established decreasing trend across sessions evident in Figure 9.1), but the pre-post changes in scores were not statistically reliable using the RCI method. There was an improvement in physical fatigue (but again not statistically reliable), and overall quality of life remained relatively stable.

Conversely, his depression scores moved reliably (an increase in symptoms) from the borderline to moderate range on the HADS, although this has been an oscillating element of his life prior to the group. Cognitive fatigue increased during the first three months of group attendance but returned to baseline levels during the second half of the group. Psychosocial fatigue remained stable and minimal throughout.

Mark's subjective experience of the TJ group was captured in these quotes from the focus group evaluation (full group findings reported in Yeates et al., submitted). He described the impact of the group on relaxation, alongside the present-moment focus of the group being a relief – there was no pressure to remember content and show others he was progressing at a comparable rate to others:

> It teaches you how to relax . . . if you can sit down and relax, it teaches you how to kind of . . . let go and slow down. . . . I feel calmer after it.
>
> There wasn't too much pressure to remember stuff like it was just the usefulness of doing the exercise in itself rather than having to learn . . . I don't seem to pick it up very much but I didn't feel that pressure that I needed to kinda progress too much. . . . I normally do I feel that I'd be letting the teacher down (in other community classes/activities) if I didn't.

Mark did struggle with increased fatigue throughout the group from the mental stimulation necessitated from getting hospital transport to travel for 45 minutes to attend the 90-minute sessions (including a break) and then return home:

> What's challenging about the actual doing the day is, for me is, the fatigue . . . with the coming in on transport, ermm they get us here very early and so it makes the day quite long and I have to sleep sort of all afternoon after it.

Mark had struggled to engage in a range of community-based leisure activities in the ten years since his injury, due the constant interplay of physical, cognitive and emotional difficulties. The TJ was an exception, and Mark managed to participate in majority of sessions within the 6-month group, despite the impact of the attendance (both session participation and the 90-minute return travel) on his fatigue (trends in his physical fatigue scale scores over time did indicate a trend for lower levels during the second half of the group). Given the constraint of fatigue, the modest trend for reduced anxiety over the course of the sessions was meaningful, again considering the enduring nature of Mark's emotional difficulties. Oscillations in low mood that characterised his life were evident throughout the course of the TJ group and were less responsive to the intervention. His comments suggest self-critical thought patterns that feature worries about letting the teacher of an activity down and comparison with other students. Here the present-moment focus of TJ offers an opportunity for mind-body development that is not linked to achievement goals or outcome – this may be one reason why he continued to attend the group and derive the anxiety reduction/relaxation/slowing down of ruminative processes benefits. He developed close friendships with other survivors in the group and found the shared mixture of progress and challenges over the course of the group for both he and others meaningful and comforting. His experience with others each week in the group stood in contrast with a socially isolated life the rest of the week. At the end of the six-month group, he was considering joining a regular TJ group in the community but was apprehensive about his progress and acceptance by others (including a new teacher).

Mark's experience shows the long-term value of TJ groups for people with enduring and complex physical, cognitive and emotional difficulties. This group was in the initial phase of the author's research, and as such was an unadapted group delivered exclusively to ABI survivors. The group as a whole included participants who benefited from significant gains in mood and fatigue as a result of attendance (Yeates, 2019, in press), and also those that did not experience any benefit or even worsened on some indices of wellbeing (Yeates et al., submitted). This underlies the aforementioned argument to include rehabilitation-based adaptations to optimise benefit from TJ practice, which will be the subject of future studies. Hopefully the potential and scope of a TJ group is evident in this case study and highlights a new paradigm for working with both mind and body in brain injury services. Finally, the need for long-term groups like TJ is also emphasised here, to be responsive to both enduring needs of survivors but also offer opportunities for aspects of functioning that may respond very slowly but steadily and positively to a new wellbeing opportunity, as evident in Mark's fatigue scores in the second three months versus the initial three months of the intervention.

Conclusions and future directions

This chapter has argued for the use of Eastern mind-body approaches as a new paradigm for simultaneous physical, psychological and spiritual support for survivors of ABI and for those with other neurological conditions. Following a brief overview of published application of yoga approaches with this clinical group, the chapter proceeded to explore Tai Ji specifically as a suitable mind-body intervention. In response to omissions within the literature, the Daoist concept of Neidan and its close counterpart in positive psychology, Flow States, have been introduced to operationalise a psychological dimension to both explain existing findings in the literature and guide the design and implementation of future TJ protocols in research to come. It is hypothesised that these suggested adaptations will increase the level of psychological (and for some, spiritual) gains from TJ practice for more people with neuro-disability. The case study offers a detailed example of the clinical value from these ideas.

Future clinical intervention research is required to evaluate the proposed TJ model in a systematic and controlled way, attending to both standardised outcome measures and subjective experience of participants. Further ideas to adapt TJ in order to optimise flow are welcome. Inherent to an evaluation of flow and its role in TJ is the need for an objective measurement methodology, both questionnaire measures and the identification of reliable physiological markers of flow state experience (such as the proposals put forward by Yeates, 2015, 2018). In anticipation of such developments, however, it is conceivable that mind-body practices used to optimise flow states may uniquely offer physical and psychological benefits for ABI survivors, an important new option given the omission of one of these elements in both physiotherapy and psychological therapy interventions within brain injury services. When explored as part of a long-term group that also confers social benefits, and one that is located in a community setting beyond the remit of short-term health services for survivors, the unique potential of a flow-based TJ group for a survivor's lifespan post-injury becomes evident.

References

Au-Yeung, S. S. Y., Hui-Chan, C. W. Y., & Tang, J. C. S. (2009). Short-form Tai Chi improves standing balance of people with chronic stroke. *Neurorehabilitation & Neural Repair, 23*, 515–522.

Bastille, J. V., & Gill-Body, K. M. (2004). A yoga-based exercise program for people with post-stroke chronic hemiparesis. *Physical Therapy, 84*, 33–48.

Blake, H., & Batson, M. (2006). Exercise intervention in brain injury: A pilot randomized study of Tai Chi Qigong. *Clinical Rehabilitation, 23*(7), 589–598.

Burschka, J. M., Keune, P. M., Oy, U., Oschman, P., & Kuhn, P. (2014). Mindfulness-based interventions in multiple sclerosis: Beneficial effects of Tai Chi on balance, coordination, fatigue and depression. *BioMedCentral Neurology, 14*(1), 165.

Chan, A. W., Sit, J. W., & Chair, S. Y. (2017). Tai Chi exercise reduces stroke risk factors: A randomized controlled trial. *Stroke, 48*, AWP416.

Csikszentmihalyi, M. (1990). *Flow: The psychology of optimal experience.* New York: Harper & Row.

Csikszentmihalyi, M. (1997). *Finding flow: The psychology of engagement with everyday life.* New York: Basic Books.

Csikszentmihalyi, M., Abuhamdeh, S., & Nakamura, J. (2005). Flow. In A. Elliot (Ed.), *Handbook of competence and motivation* (pp. 598–698). New York: Guilford Press.

Cullen, B., Pownall, J., Cummings, J., Baylan, S., Broomfield, N., Haig, C. . . . Evans, J. (2018). Positive PsychoTherapy in ABI rehab (PoPsTAR): A pilot randomised controlled trial. *Neuropsychological Rehabilitation, 28*(1), 17–33.

Damasio, A. (1999). *The feeling of what happens.* San Diego, CA: Harcourt.

Davis, B. (2004). *The Taijiquan classics: An annotated translation.* Berkeley, CA: North Atlantic.

Desrochers, P., Kairy, D., Pan, S., Corriveau, H., & Tousignant, M. (2016). Tai chi for upper limb rehabilitation in stroke patients: The patient's perspective. *Disability & Rehabilitation, 39*(13), 1313–1319.

Detert, N. (in press). Mindfulness in neurological conditions. In G. N. Yeates & F. Ashworth (Eds.), *Psychological therapies in neuropsychological rehabilitation.* Hove, UK: Psychology Press.

Ding, M. (2012). Tai Chi for stroke rehabilitation: a focused review. *American Journal of Physical Medicine & Rehabilitation, 91,* 1091–1096.

Donnelly, K. Z., Linnea, K., Grant, D. A., & Lichtenstein, J. (2014). The feasibility and impact of a yoga pilot programme on the quality-of-life of adults with acquired brain injury. *Brain Injury, 31*(2), 208–214.

Elliot, B. (2011). Arts-based and narrative inquiry in liminal experience reveal platforming as basic social psychological process. *The Arts in Psychotherapy, 38,* 96–103.

Elsass, L. & Kinsella, G. (1987). Social interaction following severe closed head injury. *Psychological Medicine, 17*(1), 67–78.

Evans, J. J. (2011). Positive psychology and brain injury rehabilitation. *Brain Impairment, 12*(2), 117–127.

Evans, J. J., & Cullen, B. (in press). Positive psychotherapy for neurological conditions. In G. N. Yeates & F. Ashworth (Eds.), *Psychological therapies in neuropsychological rehabilitation.* Hove, UK: Psychology Press.

Fisk, J. D., Ritvo, P. G., Ross, L., Haasem, D. A., Marrie, T. J., & Schlech, W. F. (1994). Measuring the functional impact of fatigue: Initial validation of the fatigue impact scale. *Clinical Infectious Disease, 18*(Supplement 1), s79–s83.

Gemmell, C., & Leathem, J. M. (2006). A study investigating the effects of tai chi chuan: Individuals with traumatic brain injury compared to controls. *Brain Injury, 20,* 151–156.

Goldstein, K. (1959). Notes on the development of my concepts. *Journal of Individual Psychology, 15,* 5–14.

Hart, J., Kanner, H., Gilboa-Mayo, R., Haroeh-Peer, O., Rozenthul-Sorokin, N., & Eldar, R. (2004). Tai Chi Chuan practice in community-dwelling persons after stroke. *International Journal of Rehabilitation Research, 27,* 303–304.

Haslam, C., Holme, A., Haslam, S. A., Lyer, A., Jetten, J., & Williams, W. H. (2008). Maintaining group memberships: social identity continuity predicts well-being after stroke. *Neuropsychological Rehabilitation, 18,* 671–691.

Hwang, I., Song, R., Ahn, S., Lee, M., Wayne, P., & Sohn, M. K. (2019). Exploring the adaptability of Tai Chi to stroke rehabilitation. *Rehabilitation Nursing, 44*(4), 221–229.

Jacobson, N. S., & Truax, P. (1991). Clinical significance: A statistical approach to defining meaningful change in psychotherapy research. *Journal of Consulting and Clinical Psychology, 59,* 12–19.

Jahnke, R., Larkey, L., Rogers, C., Etnier, J., & Lin, F. (2012). A comprehensive review of health benefits of qi gong and tai chi. *American Journal of Health Promotion, 24*(6), e1–e25.

Lazaridou, A., Philbrook, P., & Tzika, A. A. (2013). Yoga and mindfulness as therapeutic interventions for stroke rehabilitation: A systematic review. *Evidence-based Complementary and Alternative Medicine: eCAM, 2013,* 357108.

Lee, B. (2000). *Striking thoughts: Bruce Lee's wisdom for daily living.* New York: Tuttle Publishing.

Little, J., & Lee, B. (2000). *Bruce Lee: A warrior's journey.* TV Documentary. Warner Home.

Lundgren, T., Dahl, J., Yardi, N., & Melin, L. (2008). Acceptance and commitment therapy and yoga for drug-refractory epilepsy: a randomized controlled trial. *Epilepsy & Behaviour, 13,* 102–108.

Luria, A. R. (1975). *The man with a shattered world*. Harmondsworth: Penguin Books.

Lynton, H., Kligler, B., & Shiflett, S. (2007). Yoga in stroke rehabilitation: A systematic review and results of a pilot study. *Topics in Stroke Rehabilitation, 14*(4), 1–8.

Lyu, D., Lyu, X., Zhang, Y., Ren, Y., Yang, F., Zhou, L. . . . Li, Z. (2018). Tai Chi for stroke rehabilitation: A systematic review and meta-analysis of randomized controlled trials. *Frontiers in Physiology, 9*, 983. https://doi.org/10.3389/fphys.2018.00983

Moustgaard, A., Bedard, M., & Felteau, M. (2007). Mindfulness-based Cognitive Therapy (MBCT) for individuals who had a stroke: Results from a pilot 90 study. *The Journal of Cognitive Rehabilitation, 25*(4), 4–10.

Nochi, M. (1997). Dealing with the "void": Traumatic brain injury as a story. *Disability and Society, 12*, 533–555.

Nochi, M. (1998a). Struggling with the labelled self: People with traumatic brain injuries in social settings. *Qualitative Health Research, 8*, 665–681.

Nochi, M. (1998b). "Loss of self" in the narratives of people with traumatic brain injuries: A qualitative analysis. *Social Science and Medicine, 7*, 869–878.

Nochi, M. (2000). Reconstructing self-narratives in coping with traumatic brain injury. *Social Science and Medicine, 51*, 1795–1804.

Qin, L., Wei, X., Liu, L., & Zhu, H. (2016). Effectiveness of Tai Chi on movement, emotion and quality of life in patients with stroke: A Meta-analysis. *Zhongguo Zuzhi Gongcheng Yanjiu, 20*, 297–303.

Quinn, D., & Jones, K. (2012). *Tai chi movement (TMW) and embodied mindfulness in mental and physical health*. Inservice Presentation for Herefordshire Primary Care Trust, UK.

Rajesh, B., Jayachandran, D., Mohandas, G., & Radhakrishnan, K. (2006). A pilot study of a yoga meditation protocol for patients with medically refractory epilepsy. *The Journal of Alternative and Complementary Medicine, 12*(4), 367–371.

Russell, T. A. (2011). Body in mind training: Mindful movement for severe and enduring mental illness. *British Journal of Wellbeing, 2*(4), 13–16.

Russell, T. A., & Tatton-Ramos, T. (2014). Body in mind training: Mindful movement for the clinical setting. *Neuro-Disability & Psychotherapy, 2*(1/2), 108–136.

Sacks, O. (1973). *Awakenings*. New York: Random House.

Schaffer, O. (2013). *Crafting fun user experiences: A method to facilitate flow*. Human Factors International. http://humanfactors.com/downloads/whitepapers/FunExperiences.pdf

Schmidt, A. A., Miller, K. K., Van Puymbroeck, M., & Schalk, N. (2016). Feasibility and results of a case study of yoga to improve physical functioning in people with chronic traumatic brain injury. *Disability & Rehabilitation, 38*(9), 914–920.

Shapira, M. Y., Chelouche, M., Yanai, R., Kaner, C., & Szold, A. (2001). Tai Chi Chuan practice as a tool for rehabilitation of severe head trauma: 3 case reports. *Archives of Physical Medicine & Rehabilitation, 82*(9), 1283–1285.

Shravat, A. (2014). The role of a yoga group within a holistic rehabilitation setting for ABI using compassion focused therapy approach: A qualitative case illustration. *Neuro-Disability & Psychotherapy, 2*(1/2), 100–107.

Silverthorne, C., Khalsa, S. B., Gueth, R., DeAvilla, N., & Pansini, J. (2012). Respiratory, physical, and psychological benefits of breath-focused yoga for adults with severe Traumatic Brain Injury (TBI): A brief pilot study report. *International Journal of Yoga Therapy, 22*(1), 47–51.

Taylor-Piliae, R. E., Hoke, T. M., Hepworth, J. T., Latt, L. D., Najafi, B. & Coull, B. M. (2014). Effect of Tai Chi on physical function, fall rates and quality of life among older stroke survivors. *Archives of Physical Medicine and Rehabilitation 95*, 816–824.

Tyerman, A., & Humphrey, M. (1984). Changes in self concept following severe head injury. *International Journal of Rehabilitation Research, 7*, 11–23.

Wang, C., Bannuru, R., Ramel, J., Kupelnick, B., Scott, T., & Schmid, C. H. (2010). Tai Chi on psychological well-being: Systematic review and meta-analysis. *BMC Complementary Alternative Medicine, 10*, 23.

Williams, W. H., & Evans. (2003). Brain injury and emotion: an overview to a special issue on biopsychosocial approaches in neurorehabilitation. *Neuropsychological Rehabilitation, 13*(1/12), 1–11.

Wilson, B. A., Evans, J., Baddeley, A., & Shiel, A. (2010). Errorless learning in the rehabilitation of memory impaired people. *Neuropsychological Rehabilitation, 4*(3), 307–326.

Winser, S. J., Kannan, P., Pang, M., Smith, C., & Tsang, W. W. (2018). Potential benefits and safety of T'ai Chi for balance and functional independence in people with cerebellar ataxia. *The Journal of Alternative and Complimentary Medicine, 24*(12), 1221–1223.

Winser, S. J., Kannan, P., Pang, M., & Tsang, W. W. (2017). Tai chi for improving balance in cerebellar ataxia: A feasibility. *Archives of Physical Medicine & Rehabilitation, 98*(10), e113–e114.

Wu, S., Chen, J., Wang, S., Jiang, M., Wang, X., & Wen, Y. (2018). Effect of Tai Chi exercise on balance function of stroke patients: A meta-analysis. *Medical Science Monitor Basic Research, 24*, 210–215.

Xie, G. L., Rao, T., Lin, L., Lin, Z., Xiao, T., Yang, M. . . . Chen, L. (2018). Effects of Tai Chi Yunshou exercise on community-based stroke patients: A cluster randomized controlled trial. *European Review of Aging and Physical Activity, 15*, 17.

Yan Li, G., Wang, W., Liu, G. L., & Zhang, Y. (2018). Effects of Tai Chi on balance and gait in stroke survivors: A systematic meta-analysis of randomized controlled trials. *Journal of Rehabilitation Medicine, 50*(7), 582–588.

Yeates, G. N. (2014). Using pagers and alerts as adjuncts to psychological therapies following acquired brain injury. In Anna Cantagallo (Ed.), *Telerehabilitation and adaptations: assistive technology for people with neuropsychological impairments*. Milan: FrancoAngeli.

Yeates, G. N. (2015). Flow state experiences as a biopsychosocial guide for Tai Ji intervention and research in neuro-rehabilitation. *Neuro-Disability & Psychotherapy, 3*(1), 22–41.

Yeates, G.N. (2016). Neuro Flow Groups. www.neuro-flowgroup.com

Yeates, G. N. (2018). Flow state experiences as a biopsychosocial guide for Tai Ji intervention and research in neuro-rehabilitation. In G. N. Yeates & G. Farrell (Eds.), *Neuro-disability & psychotherapy, specialist topics (volume I). Eastern influences on neuropsychotherapy: Accepting, soothing and stilling cluttered and critical minds in neurological conditions*. Oxford: Routledge.

Yeates, G. N. (2019). Eastern spirituality, mind-body practices and neuro-rehabilitation. In A. Coles & J. Collicutt (Eds.), *The neurology of religion* (pp. 191–213). Cambridge: Cambridge University Press.

Yeates, G. N. (in press). The potential contribution of mind-body interventions within psychological support following aphasia: A conceptual review and case study. In G. N. Yeates & K. Meredith (Eds.), *Neuro-disability & psychotherapy, specialist topics (volume II). Psychotherapy & aphasia: Supporting emotions & relationships*. Oxford: Routledge.

Yeates, G. N., & Farrell, G. (2014). Accepting, soothing and stilling cluttered and critical minds in neurological conditions: The influence of Eastern practices. *Neuro-Disability & Psychotherapy, 2*(1/2), 1–2.

Yeates, G. N., & Farrell, G. (2018). Editors' forward. In G. N. Yeates & G. Farrell (Eds.), *Neuro-disability & psychotherapy, specialist topics (volume I). Eastern influences on neuropsychotherapy: Accepting, soothing and stilling cluttered and critical minds in neurological conditions*. Oxford: Routledge.

Yeates, G. N., Hamill, M., Sutton, L., Psaila, K., Mohamed, S., & O'Dell, J. (2008). Dysexecutive problems and interpersonal relating following frontal brain injury: reformulation in cognitive-analytic therapy. *Neuropsychoanalysis*, 10, 43–58.

Yeates, G. N., Murphy, M., Baldwin, J., Wilkes, J., & Mahadevan, M. (2015). A pilot evaluation of a yoga group for survivors of acquired brain injury in a community setting. *Clinical Psychology Forum*, *267*, 46–51.

Yeates, G. N., Nagrani, S., Smith, A., Dorney-Savage, J., Whitman, J., & Khan, E. (submitted). Diversity of needs in tai chi (taiji) group interventions following acquired brain injury: A mixed methods study.

Zhang, L., Layne, C., Lowder, T., & Liu, J. (2012). A review focused on the psychological effectiveness of Tai Chi on different populations. *Evidence-based Complementary & Alternative Medicine*, *2012*, 678107.

Zigmond, A. S., & Snaith, R. P. (1983). The hospital anxiety and depression scale. *Acta Psychiatrica Scandinavica*, *67*, 361–370.

Zou, L., Wang, C., Chen, X., & Wang, H. (2018). Baduanjin exercise for stroke rehabilitation: A systematic review with meta-analysis of randomized controlled trials. *International Journal of Environmental Research & Public Health*, *15*, 600.

Zou, L., Yeung, A., Zeng, N., Wang, C., Sun, L., Thomas, G., & Wang, H. (2018). Effects of mind-body exercises for mood and functional capabilities in post-stroke patients: An analytical review of randomized controlled trials. *International Journal of Environmental Research & Public Health*, *15*, 721.

10

INTEGRATIVE PSYCHOTHERAPY FOR HOLISTIC NEUROREHABILITATION

Pamela Klonoff and Erin Piper

Definition of integrative psychotherapy

Integrative psychotherapy denotes incorporating eclectic approaches rather than being wedded to a single theoretical orientation (Zarbo, Tasca, Cattafi, & Compare, 2016). Integrative psychotherapy encompasses theoretical integration (i.e., creating a single approach using assorted models); technical eclecticism (i.e., taking effective ingredients from diverse styles); assimilative integration (i.e., using one model but integrating components of others, as needed); and the common factors approach (i.e., emphasising applicable therapeutic practices shared within a multiplicity of methods) (Zarbo et al., 2016). Integrative psychotherapy presupposes a link between theory, evidence and technique (Norcross & Goldfried, 2005).

The theoretical application of integrated psychotherapy to neurological populations

Rehabilitation psychology's emphasis on interdisciplinary perspectives lends itself nicely to an amalgam of theoretical methodologies (Dunn & Elliot, 2008). To that end, this chapter will demonstrate how integrative psychotherapy has rich application to psychotherapy for patients after acquired brain injury (ABI). Pertinent schools of thought include psychodynamic constructs, self-psychology, behavioural modification, behaviour therapy, cognitive behavioural therapy, psychoeducation and skills training, family systems and schema, psychopharmacology, assistive technology, grief and bereavement therapy, existential psychology, Acceptance and Commitment Therapy (ACT) and mindfulness, narrative therapy and positive psychology (Brunner, Hemsley, Togher, & Palmer, 2017; Klonoff, 2010, 2014; Ruff & Chester, 2014; Wiart, Luauté, Stefan, Plantier, & Hamonet, 2016). Autobiographical books and articles as well as group interventions for patients and their support networks are vital accompaniments. Helpful group venues include cognitive reha-bilitation and group psychotherapy for patients and a family group for the support network (Klonoff, 2010, 2014).

'Common factors' in integrative psychotherapy in a holistic milieu-oriented setting enables patients with ABI the opportunity to heighten their awareness (i.e., knowledge of their ABI-related strengths and difficulties), acceptance (i.e., coping mechanisms with implementation of an armamentarium of compensa-tions) and realism (i.e., making solid judgments for the future), define their post-injury identity and create a purposeful existence (Klonoff, 2010; Wiart et al., 2016). Proven 'common factors' for successful outcomes include a cohesive team working synchronously with each other, patients, families and 'tiers of support' community supporters, addressing patients' many needs in a nurturing 'safe haven' milieu environment and fostering a fortified working alliance (Klonoff, 2010, 2014; Schönberger, Humle, & Teasdale, 2006; Vestri et al., 2014).

Integrative psychotherapy also addresses post-injury functioning holistically, employing the emotional, interpersonal, cognitive, language, physical, functional, quality of life and spiritual domains. It takes into account patients' (and caregivers') unique pre-injury psychodynamic, historical, developmental, personality, cul-tural, motivational, aspirational, value-based and environmental considerations. Techniques are predicated on structure, accountability, proper timing and pacing of feedback, collateral data and empathic guidance (Elliott, Bohart, Watson, & Murphy, 2018; Klonoff, 2010). Regular note-taking on integral ideas, journaling and integration of 'rehab lingo', slogans, mantras, metaphors, diagrams, drawings, exercises and complementary media all improve the psychotherapeutic effective-ness by reaching the patient in his or her phenomenological world (Klonoff, 2010, 2014).

Evidence-based research on integrated psychotherapy for patients with ABI

Evidence-based research on integrative psychotherapy for patients with ABI is relatively sparse but is developing. Fang, Mpofu, and Athanasou (2017) applied a constructive integrative psychosocial intervention (i.e., psychoeducation, narra-tives, problem solving, crisis management and activity participation) with a con-sequent decrease in depressive and anxiety symptoms in stroke survivors. Other studies have highlighted ways to optimise patients' psychosocial and functional outcomes (i.e., productive work and driving) based on key therapeutic entities (e.g., a positive working alliance) (Klonoff et al., 2010; Martelli, Zasler, & Tiernan, 2012) as well as with comprehensive, interdisciplinary, holistic methods (Cattelani, Zettin, & Zoccolotti, 2010; Cicerone et al., 2011; Martelli et al., 2012). 'Com-mon factor' research variables that enhance learning contain errorless learning, task analysis and graduated exposure (Martelli et al., 2012). Overall, however, more research is needed to address uncontrolled variables with rigorous inclusion/exclusion criteria and clear specification of the theoretical basis, design and treat-ment contents (Cattelani et al., 2010).

The practical application of integrative psychotherapy for individuals with ABI

Deciding upon psychotherapy practices is a fluid craft, yet sometimes it is daunting. These authors posit first investigating 'precursor' factors, which are contextual and on a broad spectrum. As clinical or rehabilitation psychologists, the practitioner requires extensive knowledge in brain and behaviour relationships based on scientific and clinical vigor (Dunn & Elliott, 2008). This provides an umbrella for the intricacies of neurological damage and usually wide-ranging consequences. For example, patients with severe aphasia may be best suited for cognitive behavioural therapy and basic psychoeducation, rather than highly abstract, language-based interventions (e.g., narrative or existential therapies).

'Individualised' considerations are also essential, within the psychotherapist, patient, support network and treatment setting. These set the stage for further customisation and refinement. Case in point, the psychotherapist's training, theoretical orientation(s), preferences, clinical experience and skill set (or lack thereof) will shape the choices, course and outcomes of therapy. Schooling and know-how with various modalities, such as individual versus group interventions, are also pertinent. Conversely, the relative presence and weightings of possible neurological 'precursor' limitations (be they physical, cognitive, emotional, behavioural, interpersonal, functional, etc.) in combination with the unique perturbations of each individual's and his or her family's pre- and post-injury life experiences will influence how the integrative psychotherapy process unfolds. Therefore, the clinician should always obtain relevant personalised information, including medical records delineating the nature and course of the patient's ABI, neuropsychological test findings and interview data concerning the patient's particular background demographics, social history, developmental and educational variables and occupational history (Klonoff, 2010). The patient's and support network's personalised subjective renditions of their post-injury condition are also important, including the physical, cognitive/language, emotional and interpersonal impairments, family relationships, hobbies and leisure interests and community integration aspirations (e.g., work or school). Finally, and notably, the healthcare system opportunities and constraints impact psychotherapeutic methods.

Together, these 'precursor' and 'individualised' factors inform the rich interplay of the facets of the individual's current psychological makeup, which serves as a blueprint for optimal integrative psychotherapy choices. Figure 10.1 is an illustration of subcomponents of integrative psychotherapy in a holistic milieu neurorehabilitation environment. Using this theoretical formulation, this chapter will illustrate integrative psychotherapy in a holistic milieu environment using two clinical typologies: moderate to severe brain injuries at a young age (age 16 or less) and patients who were high-level professionals and gifted preinjury. 'Precursor' considerations applicable to pre-determinations of integrative psychotherapy practices will be presented, followed by "individualised" integrative psychotherapy methods employing case study material.

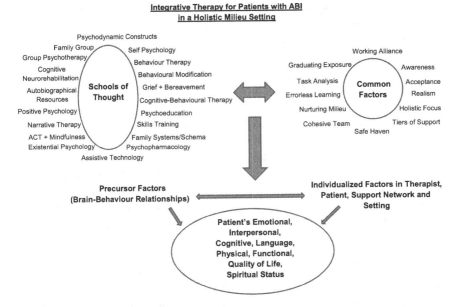

**Integrative Therapy for Patients with ABI
in a Holistic Milieu Setting**

Psychodynamic Constructs

Family Group

Group Psychotherapy

Cognitive
Neurorehabilitation

Autobiographical
Resources

Positive Psychology

Narrative Therapy

ACT + Mindfulness

Existential Psychology

Assistive Technology

Self Psychology

Behaviour Therapy

Behavioural Modification

**Schools of
Thought**

Grief + Bereavement

Cognitive-Behavioural Therapy

Psychoeducation

Skills Training

Family Systems/Schema

Psychopharmacology

Working Alliance

Graduating Exposure

Task Analysis

Errorless Learning

Nurturing Milieu

Cohesive Team

Awareness

**Common
Factors**

Acceptance

Realism

Holistic Focus

Tiers of Support

Safe Haven

Precursor Factors
(Brain-Behaviour Relationships)

Individualized Factors in Therapist,
Patient, Support Network and
Setting

Patient's Emotional,
Interpersonal,
Cognitive, Language,
Physical, Functional,
Quality of Life,
Spiritual Status

FIGURE 10.1   Integrative therapy for patients with ABI in a holistic milieu setting

Integrative psychotherapy for patients with ABI at a young age

Pre-treatment "precursor" considerations

The backdrop in the pre-planning phase of integrative psychotherapy for individuals sustaining brain injuries at a young age is an understanding of normal development as well as concomitant interruptions after brain injury. Reasons are the presence or absence of: (1) predispositions to acquired brain injury (e.g., Attention Deficit and Hyperactivity Disorder and psychosocial adversity [Schachar, Park, & Dennis, 2015]); and (2) the relative severity and location of the brain injury, given that social functioning, life challenges, outcome and quality of life are worse for youngsters with more severe diffuse and focal damage, especially involving the frontal lobes and corpus callosum (Di Battista, Soo, Catroppa, & Anderson, 2012; Rosema, Crowe, & Anderson, 2012). Critical is the realisation of the 'theory of vulnerability', which suggests that earlier brain injuries affect the developing brain more (Li & Liu, 2012), and that brain damage often results in "arrested development" (Ewing-Cobbs et al., 2008).

Major pre-treatment "precursors" that shape interventions for youths with ABI are the typical cognitive consequences (e.g., impaired attention, language, intellect, memory, speed of thinking and executive functions [Beauchamp & Anderson, 2013]) and subsequent pervasive academic problems (Gabbe et al., 2014). With a potential ratio of one teacher to hundreds of students at school, there is a dearth of insights about and accommodations for neurological disability, and inflated aspirations in the student, parents and school personnel also associated with a lack of recognising how ABI interfaces with the 'real world'.

Post-injury personality alterations are prevalent, often manifested as internalising (e.g., anxiety, depression and low self-esteem) and externalising (e.g., hyperactivity, aggressiveness, conduct and oppositional-defiant disorders, as well as poor social communication) challenges (Li & Liu, 2012; Ryan et al., 2013). Depression frequently translates to limitations in activities, lost opportunities, loneliness, and grief and loss (Di Battista, Godfrey, Soo, Catroppa, & Anderson, 2014; Rosema et al., 2012). Social dysfunction in the forms of exclusion and rejection promulgates maladaptive behaviour, reduced self-regulation, fewer friendships and low social cognition (e.g., reduced emotion perception, social competence, social problem solving and communication pragmatics) (Rosema et al., 2012; Ryan et al., 2013). Owing to ostracism, bullying and stigmatisation at school, these participants wrestle with social marginalisation and isolation, often for the long haul (Rosema et al., 2015).

Unlike adults with ABI, a distinctive 'precursor' for youngsters with ABI is disruptions in their moral development, defined as a code of values and conduct, including empathy, gratitude, a sense of fairness, feelings of reciprocity, consolation, righteousness and group loyalty (Mendez, 2009; Pascual, Rodrigues, & Gallardo-Pujol, 2013). Subcomponents include the capacity for guilt, shame, compassion, humility, pride, fear of negative evaluation, strong motivators and decisions about right and wrong (Marazziti, Baroni, Landi, Ceresoli, & Dell'Osso, 2013; Mendez, 2009). Compounding the risk of interpersonal hurdles is the discovery that the neuroanatomy of moral behaviour overlaps with neuroanatomical locations in ABI (e.g., frontal and subcortical areas) (Mendez, 2009; Pascual et al., 2013). Moreover, a biology x environmental interaction can emerge between early prefrontal lesions and detrimental peer and caregiver relations (e.g., attachment issues). This results in a failure to build appropriate scaffolding for the child's moral development (Taber-Thomas et al., 2014).

Other noteworthy theoretical antecedents to decreased honesty and integrity in this population are elements of personality disorders, due to the nature of traumatic events and early age disturbances in perception, speed of information processing, affect and internal controls causing dysfunctional beliefs (i.e., schemas) and maladaptive strategies (Beck, 2014). For instance, antisocial personality disorder characteristics identified in these patients (with a frontal syndrome) included impulsivity, verbal and physical aggressiveness and pervasively irresponsible behaviour; a self-view of feeling victimised by society; an attitude of entitlement to break rules; overdeveloped strategies of manipulation, deception and thrill seeking and underdeveloped strategies of empathy, rule adherence and behavioural inhibition (Beck, 2014; Tomaszewski et al., 2014).

Aspects of a narcissistic personality disorder can emerge, including a self-perception of being special and entitled to favourable attentiveness, feeling above the rules, an underlying covert belief that he or she is unlovable and helpless, overdeveloped strategies of transcending rules and ordinary limits and under-developed strategies of showing empathy and consideration, inhibiting impulses and social reciprocity (Beck, 2014). Hypothetically, socialisation influences are invoked in moral development. 'Moral agency' emerges from moral failures in combination with social input (e.g., the mother's guidance) and cultural norms, which then affects moral development and expression (Lapsley & Carlo, 2014).

Another salient context is the 'precursor' family factors caused by the brain injury aftermath. Demographic risk, including difficulties with finances, mater-nal mental health, parenting interactions and resilience, as well as low parenting morale, intensify the child's behavioural issues (Cabaj, McDonald, & Tough, 2014). Maladaptive parenting modes, inadequate family cohesion, parental dis-tress, mediocre awareness, permissiveness (e.g., less supervision and structure), low socioeconomic status and lack of a parent leader negatively affect outcomes after brain injury in youth after ABI, including self-regulation and other execu-tive functions (Li & Liu, 2012; Rosema et al., 2012).

'Precursor' clinical presentation and integrative psychotherapy treatment formulations

Based on early clinical observations and assessment in the neurorehabilitation environment, this cohort of youth with ABI present with broad-spectrum 'pre-cursor' behavioural, emotional and communication pragmatic challenges. These are characterised by immaturity, deficient self-regulation (e.g., impulsivity and insufficient safety awareness) and depleted social skills, manifested as being clingy, overbearing, shy and/or withdrawn. Mood symptoms are widespread, including depression (e.g., sleep disturbance, low energy, social withdrawal, low self-esteem, self-deprecation, apathy, guilt, lack of drive, joy, and pleasure, hope-lessness, helplessness and worthlessness), fear and anxiety, easy embarrassment, irritability ('snarkiness') and catastrophic reactions (CRs) (Goldstein, 1952).

'Unprofessional behaviour', especially in group settings, and disinhibited social and sexual behaviour abound. Dishonest, risky and naïve behaviours are evident in accordance with arrested development, also morally. With a 1:1 staff-patient ratio in the neurorehabilitation environment, patients (and families) grapple with perceiv-ing oversight in the neurorehabilitation environment as 'micromanaging' compared to the 'hands off' manner at school. A sheltered view of reality results in early scepticism towards therapy recommendations by both patients and their relatives.

Thus, foundational to any potential movement in psychotherapy, regardless of the technique, is establishment of rapport-building through the 'common fac-tors' approach of empathic attunement with a cocreated experience, an open lis-tening stance, collaborative partnership, 'meeting the patient where he or she is' and gentle and timely interpretations fostering self-understanding (Elliott et al., 2018; Klonoff, 2010; Wolf, 1988).

Multidimensional integrative 'technical eclecticism' methodologies can be merged, including behaviour therapy, cognitive behavioural therapy and psycho-education and skills training on social and age-appropriate interactions (in both individual and group formats). Due to mood and behavioural issues, supplemental psychopharmacology through close collaboration with a psychiatrist sets the stage for greater embracement of therapeutic suggestions. Group psychotherapy promotes didactics and deep peer dialogue about the tribulations of neurorehabilitation and recovery.

Functionally, cognitive deficits and developmental delays produce a slow learning curve in adopting compensations. There is meager detail in note-taking in the datebook and fluctuating scores on a structured format to complete home chores (i.e., the Home Independence Checklist [HIC]; Klonoff, 2010). They have difficulty with problem solving and setting priorities (e.g., doing homework versus attending social events). An enduring theme is to frame therapeutic expectations as 'work ready' behaviours, through accountability and integrity training, as these individuals are inevitably hungry to drive and work. This includes 'theoretical integration' of cognitive rehabilitation, skill building through modelling and guidance by older milieu peers and therapists, implementing 'Professional Behaviours' logs with specific 'do's' and 'avoids' for proper self-monitoring of communication pragmatics and placing patients on 'probationary status' with specific contingencies to be eligible for program participation and eventual work and school endeavours (Klonoff, 2010). Self-psychology principles are extracted for corrective emotional experiences through good self-object experiences, empathic attunement and positive mirroring and idealising transference relationships. This regulates self-esteem, develops self-discipline and creates self-worth, inner resiliency and psychological wellbeing (Klonoff, 2014; Kohut, 1984). Mindfulness and ACT constructs infuse a value-driven existence and help patients envision a meaningful and fulfilled future (Hayes, Strosahl, & Wilson, 2003; Pollak, Pedulla, & Siegel, 2016).

Another "precursor" factor is that considerable family dysfunction from the long-term ramifications of an early life brain injury on the siblings, parents and other relatives is 'the norm'. Often there is 'skewed' attention to the loved one, to the exclusion of other relatives. 'Burn out' and 'compassion fatigue' (Klonoff, 2014) are pervasive. The stated expectation is that the individual will 'catch up' developmentally, cognitively and socially, with the neurorehabilitation expected to 'work miracles' in this regard. Integrative psychotherapy targets family psychoeducation and builds awareness, acceptance and realism, also using instructional materials (e.g., the Patient Experiential Model of Recovery [PEM]; the Family Experiential Model of Recovery [FEM]); as well as other didactics and readings (Klonoff, 2010, 2014; Winson, Wilson, & Bateman, 2017).

Useful formats are individual meetings with family members, conjoint sessions with their loved one, attendance at a weekly family group and joining forces with other interdisciplinary team members for general education on ABI and compensation training (Klonoff, 2014). Fortification of a mutually sturdy, culturally sensitive working alliance and common view of therapeutic principles and goals are crucial for any progress with the loved one (Klonoff, 2014). This includes the relatives' willingness to provide sufficient supervision at home and in the community and their commitment to assisting the loved one with home tasks (e.g., medication management, as well as usage of datebook and checklist systems). Mindfulness, positive psychology and ACT concepts are valuable in breeding self-reflection, self-care and a hopeful outlook in the support network.

Case study of a patient with ABI at a young age: 'individualised' integrative psychotherapy

Pre-treatment 'precursor' considerations

Ruth was a 19-year-old status-post medulloblastoma resection at age 10 with subsequent radiation and chemotherapy, consistent with vulnerable brain development. Her physiatrist wanted Ruth rehabilitated to a competitive employment position. Contextual 'precursor' considerations included expected impaired balance, coordination and fine motor challenges, memory and attention impairments and significant executive dysfunction, indicating the undeniable link between the cerebellum and prefrontal circuits (Bodranghien et al., 2016).

'Individualised' clinical presentation and integrative treatment formulations and interventions

Ruth's 'personalised' medical records highlighted a dearth of any outpatient therapies and resultant psychosocial antecedents of poor grades, school bullying, depression and friendlessness, a fractured home life and job terminations due to deceitful behaviour.

Early clinical observations in the neurorehabilitation milieu revealed Ruth's 'individualised' factors of poor communication pragmatics, including entrenched difficulties with self-centredness, turn-taking, disinhibition and snarkiness. She displayed antisocial characteristics of undependable behaviour, deception and rule breaking. Her immaturity, excuse-making and poor judgment signified her arrested development.

The "common factors" emphasis was to fortify a working alliance between Ruth and her interdisciplinary team and then inculcate an awareness and acceptance of her ABI-related sequelae, with embracement of vital tools to serve realistic and attainable goals. 'Technical eclecticism' and 'assimilative integration' integrative psychotherapy methods employed individual and group psychotherapy venues and adjunct psychiatric treatment. PEM psychoeducation and skills training stimulated Ruth's use of a personalised datebook and HIC to account for her memory and attention challenges and executive dysfunction. After seeking specialised training in developmental psychology, the psychotherapist helped Ruth develop 'Golden Rules' (e.g., be sensitive to the needs of others, listen more, avoid excuse making, avoid negotiating, take notes and avoid finding loopholes) and a 'Professional Behaviours' log, both of which provided a behaviour modification rubric and instantaneous feedback about moral transgressions. A work-like 'probationary status' was implemented to coach accountability. This was supplemented with essay writing and teachings on fundamental moral principles, such as integrity, respect and gratitude. Psychiatric expertise proffered a mood stabiliser to reduce impulsivity.

Guided and empathic exploration using ACT and existential constructs to address her deep underlying depression and angst vis a vis the future, and cognitive behavioural therapy to advance healthier coping skills, including tackling anger management and assertiveness workbooks, all mended her mood disorder. Eventually, heartfelt sharing about cyberbullying and social alienation in the safe haven of group psychotherapy, in combination with didactics and other patients' input on establishing new friendships forged first-time meaningful bonds with peers. Pre-meditated script writing and role play exercises in a social skills group foreshadowed healthy community social forays. Career exploration, mock interviews and mentoring by a former patient with a similar ABI background, now thriving in a 'first-step' 'right fit' job, softened Ruth's preoccupation with unrealistic paths. Empathic attunement through mirroring and idealising transferences with her psychotherapist in a nurturing milieu simulated 're-raising' Ruth through developmental and moral milestones, resulting in a cohesive sense of self.

Ruth's high achieving parents (i.e., a prominent lawyer and prosperous accountant) refused to accept their daughter as 'disabled'. Maladaptive parenting (e.g., overindulgence), marital discord; and rigid and unrealistic expectations concerning Ruth's functionality and employment resulted in all parties displaying 'pie in the sky' ambitions, despite her abysmal academic and employment history. Ruth's behavioural outbursts and poor social choices necessitated 24/7 supervision at home with all parties feeling 'imprisoned' by her ABI. Feeling 'micro-managed', her parents avoided attending scheduled psychotherapy appointments and a 'common factors' analysis exposed a stalled working alliance.

Clinical delving revealed that Ruth's parents were consumed with distrust and fearfulness. A 'technical eclecticism' orientation facilitated an exploration of feelings of 'ambiguous loss', "chronic sorrow', 'loss spirals' and grief styles (intuitive versus instrumental) through private and family group sessions. This enabled 'companioning' with the psychotherapist and other beleaguered families (Roos, 2002). Using family systems therapy, (Kreutzer, Marwitz, Godwin, & Arango-Lasprilla, 2010), Ruth's parents revealed their underlying cycle of shame and self-recriminations about their daughter's 'defectiveness'. Ways to mitigate 'symbiotic enmeshment' (Roos, 2002) and CRs by proxy (Klonoff, 2014) were explored through 're-parenting' self-psychology techniques of 'optimal frustration' and 'transmuting internalization' so as to reconstruct Ruth's ego structure

(Wolf, 1988). Marital counseling rebalanced boundaries; Ruth matriculated from a regressed 'center of her family's universe' to a healthy synergetic adult daughter role. Together, Ruth and her parents started weekly 'milieu meetings' (Klonoff, 2010). This review of family business, progress and concerns created harmony and reinforced trustworthy and mature behaviour.

Outcome

Through integrative psychotherapy, Ruth's parents' outward hostile stance shifted to self-forgiveness, 'letting go' and illumination of a hopeful path towards future triumphs and happiness. Via evolved awareness, acceptance and realism, Ruth and her parents now championed the concept of 'a job' versus 'the job'. After several growth-promoting interviews, she obtained a part-time position at a local library, sorting and checking out books, which was consonant with her aptitudes and interests. Therapists (including her psychotherapist) accompanied her initially for moral support and to aid her in incorporating the necessary strategies to ensure success. Healthy family dynamics prevailed; Ruth enjoyed new freedoms, including unsupervised time at home whilst her parents took short rejuvenating vacations.

Collaboration with a Recreational Therapist addressed Ruth's ongoing loneliness and social ostracism. She was introduced to healthy social outlets, through a church singles group and a brain injury social group. As Ruth eased out of the holistic milieu environment, she vocalised at her graduation (i.e., 'cake day', Klonoff, 2010), an appreciation for her psychotherapist 'sticking by her side despite some of her earlier antics and struggles, and even after she let out [her] true colors, a.k.a. [her] bad habits'. She acknowledged that although her rehabilitation took 'two long, hard years', she viewed it as a 'godsend'. She also maturely credited her unfolding positive sense of self, enhanced independence, genuine satisfaction and life meaning to her parents' backing.

Integrative psychotherapy for higher level professional and gifted patients

Pre-treatment 'precursor' considerations

Integrative psychotherapy can be especially beneficial for high functioning and talented individuals who suffer brain injuries and cannot easily return to their premorbid capabilities, including domain-general targets that support learning, adaptation and cognition and energy to cultivate effortful and goal-directed behaviour (Chen & Loya, 2014). Germane pre-treatment 'precursor' variables are the estimates of 'self-relative' cognitive and language faculties as well as 'brain reserve'/'cognitive reserve capacity', pervasiveness of higher order executive function deficits and alterations in their sense of self and identity.

Self-relative estimates of the individual's performance prior to the ABI combats the 'diluting comparison factor', whereby post-injury capabilities are targeted at the 'average range' or 'middle of the pack' (Lanham & Misukanis, 1999; Lezak, Howieson, Loring, Hannay, & Fischer, 2004). As examples, scores in the normatively average range for patients who premorbidly operated in the superior range are considered a mild self-relative deficit, whilst scores in the normatively mildly impaired range are considered a severe self-relative impairment. 'Brain reserve' (i.e., the amount of brain damage that can be sustained before it reaches a threshold of clinical expression) and 'cognitive reserve capacity' (i.e., higher intelligence as well as educational and occupational feats) are mechanisms to augment recovery in this population (Bigler & Stern, 2015). Another pre-treatment 'precursor' is the risk and dire upshots of executive dysfunction on home and community independence (Dodson, 2010; Klonoff, 2010, 2014). Universally, there are also crushing effects on one's sense of self, identity and social roles (Klonoff, 2010).

'Precursor' clinical presentation and integrative psychotherapy treatment formulations

Early clinical observations in the neurorehabilitation environment indicate these professional and gifted patients experience overwhelming angst concerning the uncertainty of their futures, both with respect to reclaiming their work and societal standing as well as their financial stability. This regularly leads to considerable depression, anxiety, narcissistic rage and CRs (Klonoff, 2010).

Requisite 'common factors' approaches entail empathic responsiveness, or 'looking out his or her (sometimes bleak) window as a fellow traveler' (Yalom, 2002); entering the patient's 'lived space' (Fuchs, 2007), also by learning about his or her 'job lingo'; promoting optimal awareness, acceptance and realism employing concepts such as errorless learning; and analysis of duties as an 'information broker', especially in complex vocational realms (Dodson, 2010). Frequent objectives are graduating exposure to purposeful pre-accident undertakings or identifying alternate worthwhile past-times. Multidimensional 'technical eclecticism' methods for this population include the retraining of metacognitive abilities and interpersonal skills through structured cognitive rehabilitation exercises; self-ratings of cognitive, communication, behavioural and mood impairments caused by frontal lobe damage and disrupted executive functions; group psychoeducation about the brain and recovery; and compensation instruction that is ecologically validated and generalises to the 'real world', especially employment (Chen & Loya, 2014; Dodson, 2010; Douglas, Bracy, & Snow, 2016; Klonoff, 2014). Therapist-monitored unpaid work activities constitute an invaluable steppingstone and tool for self-reflection and identity reformulation.

Emotional healing through individual and group integrative psychotherapy include grief and bereavement therapy, existential psychotherapy, narrative therapy, ACT and mindfulness and positive psychology, all of which can ameliorate the 'acceptance crisis' and 'shattering of their assumptive world' (Kauffman, 2002; Klonoff, 2010) and catalyse a 'new normal'.

Case study of a high functioning and gifted patient: 'individualised' integrative psychotherapy

Pre-treatment 'precursor' considerations

Sylvia, a 30-year-old second generation Chinese female, sustained a work-related traumatic brain injury (TBI) when she was T-boned on the driver's side by an intoxicated man. A CT scan of her head indicated the presence of a subarachnoid hemorrhage predominantly involving the left anterior frontal lobe near the convexity. Known as a highly intelligent and talented art therapist, concerns included possible executive function, verbal memory, speed of information processing and attention sequelae in the context of likely above average intelligence and the potential for a better recovery because of her brain reserve/cognitive reserve capacity. A difficult navigation through her functional and emotional tumult was anticipated.

'Individualised' clinical presentation and integrative treatment formulations and interventions

Indeed, Sylvia's intake neuropsychological testing estimated her pre-injury functioning in the superior range, with self-relative mild deficits in her verbal learning and recall (i.e., 28th–72nd percentile) and self-relative moderate difficulties (i.e., 17th–27th percentile) in selected aspects of her executive functions (i.e., novel reasoning and multitasking). Fortunately, she demonstrated preserved basic attention, speed of thinking, language (i.e., word fluency, auditory and reading comprehension, communication pragmatics and writing) and other executive functions (i.e., planning and organisation).

Sylvia (and her husband) gravitated easily to psychoeducation on TBI (especially executive function manifestations of frontal lobe damage) and compensation training. She actively embraced various tools (e.g., a datebook and the HIC). Fortunately, due to Sylvia's 'cognitive reserve capacity', she demonstrated a rapid improvement in her cognition. Remarkably, and attributable to her 'brain reserve', she maintained her clinical perceptiveness and artistic aptitude. At the time of the injury, Sylvia was married and had a son age seven. Early psychotherapy discussions also utilised ACT to explore her key values, which centred on her family and the intrinsic joy of helping troubled adolescents using art therapy.

Employing the 'common factors' style of an 'information broker'/liaison, within three months her psychotherapist facilitated Sylvia's incremental return to work. Despite graduating exposure to job demands, Sylvia had to disentangle over-identification with her clients, as she too felt 'helplessly wounded'. In a shared 'lived space' as psychotherapists, possible psychodynamic elements of counter-transference relationships in Sylvia unfurled. 'Theoretical integration' enabled an analysis of countertransference articles in the fields of neurorehabilitation and sand play (Cunningham, 2011; Klonoff, 2011). This produced healthier boundaries and also served as complementary cognitive rehabilitation and retraining of Sylvia's metacognitive skills.

Despite her many achievements, however, there remained a dampening of Sylvia's inner spirit or exuberance for life. There was a pervasive dysphoric 'blah' and bleakness that seemed impenetrable. One day, she brought some artwork she had done; it was 'discarded' in the bottom of her backpack (see Figure 10.2).

Sylvia was invited to share this; it spawned an untold conversation. Per her wispy, faceless character, she described not feeling completely present, also during her psychotherapy sessions. Sylvia wrote:

> *Misplaced time*: Holding on and letting go, together, but separated, dually allowing for inner growth and further insights. The solitude of letting go of solid parts of my identity and disillusioned concept of self, becoming lighter and closer to the true inner version of myself. Holding on to memory of life experiences, while shedding the layers of emotional packaging. Misplaced in the shadows, being in the "wrong place at the wrong time," allowed trauma and loss to soak into my heart of being and opened eyes to the light seeping in.

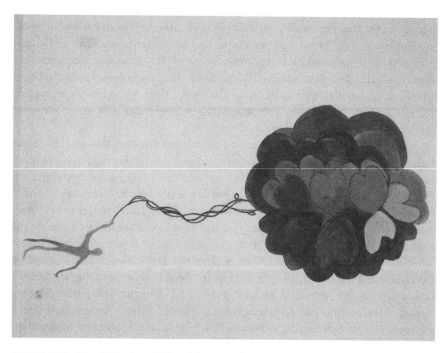

FIGURE 10.2 The 'Misplaced Time' drawing by Sylvia

Outcome

Sylvia's own artwork symbolised her anguish concerning an untold compound trauma due to the death of her baby of Sudden Infant Death Syndrome, which occurred a year (almost to the day) before her TBI. 'Theoretical integrative' psychotherapy methodologies were fused, including narrative therapy and grief and bereavement counseling. Concepts included 'why me', 'what if's', regrets, (self-) punishment and 'complicated grief' (Worden, 2009). Through psychiatric consultation, Sylvia started sertraline to ease her depressive symptoms. In accordance with her Buddhist religion, *The Book of Joy* (Dalai Lama, Tutu, & Abrams, 2016) was introduced as a culturally relevant 'roadmap' to reduce her despair. Mindfulness material, including *Full Catastrophe Living* (Kabat-Zinn, 2013) also assisted Sylvia in her emotional reconstruction. Conjoint therapy with her husband, a loving ally, fortified Sylvia during this turbulent journey and reinforced self-care and quality family time as sacred priorities.

Exploration of excerpts from *Option B* (Sandberg & Grant, 2017), and a positive psychology You-Tube video (www.youtube.com/watch?v=1qJvS8v0TTI) in group psychotherapy deeply resonated with her seemingly twisted life course. She discovered tangible ways to foster resiliency, new hope and movement from a victim to a survivor. Courageously, thanks to the nurturing ambience, she chose to share her drawing in group psychotherapy, receiving peer validation and accolades for the global and bonding messages. With a mutual fascination in art therapy, Sylvia brought many drawings to future psychotherapy sessions, all of which symbolised healing of her inner suffering. Her energy and life-force were reviving.

Conclusion

Eclectic integrative psychotherapy interventions, including a 'common factors' approach, facilitates emotional and life reconstitution for patients with varying antecedents and after-effects of ABI. 'Precursor' contextual brain-behaviour variables in combination with the 'individualised' symptom presentation of each patient (and his or her support network) in tandem with the therapist's expertise in a holistic milieu environment will drive the best psychotherapeutic modalities to effect positive growth.

References

Beauchamp, M. H., & Anderson, V. (2013). Cognitive and psychopathological sequelae of pediatric traumatic brain injury. *Handbook of Clinical Neurology, 112*, 913–920.

Beck, A. T. (2014). Theory of personality disorders. In A. T. Beck, D. D. Davis, & A. Freeman (Eds.), *Cognitive therapy of personality disorders* (3rd ed., pp. 19–6). New York: Guilford Press.

Bigler, E. D., & Stern, Y. (2015). Traumatic brain injury and reserve. *Handbook of Clinical Neurology, 128*, 691–710.

Bodranghien, F., Bastian, A., Casali, C., Hallett, M., Louis, E. D., Manto, M. . . . van Dun, K. (2016). Consensus paper: Revisiting the symptoms and signs of cerebellar syndrome. *Cerebellum, 15*(3), 369–391.

Brunner, M., Hemsley, B., Togher, L., & Palmer, S. (2017). Technology and its role in rehabilitation for people with cognitive-communication disability following a Traumatic Brain Injury (TBI). *Brain Injury, 31*(8), 1028–1043.

Cabaj, J. L., McDonald, S. W., & Tough, S. C. (2014). Early childhood risk and resilience factors for behavioural and emotional problems in middle childhood. *BMC Pediatrics, 14*, 166–176.

Cattelani, R., Zettin, M., & Zoccolotti, P. (2010). Rehabilitation treatments for adults with behavioral and psychosocial disorders following acquired brain injury: A systematic review. *Neuropsychology Review, 20*(1), 52–85.

Chen, A. J., & Loya, F. (2014). Mild-moderate TBI: Clinical recommendations to optimize neurobehavioral functioning, learning, and adaptation. *Seminars in Neurology, 34*(5), 557–571.

Cicerone, K. D., Langenbahn, D. M., Braden, C., Malec, J. F., Kalmar, K., Frass, M. . . . Ashman, T. (2011). Evidence-based cognitive rehabilitation: Updated review of the literature from 2003 through 2008. *Archives of Physical Medicine and Rehabilitation, 92*(4), 519–530.

Cunningham, L. (2011). Countertransference in sandplay: The heart and the mind of a loving, attuned other. *Journal of Sandplay Therapy, 20*(1).

Dalai Lama, Tutu, D., & Abrams, D. (2016). *The book of joy: Lasting happiness in a changing world.* New York: Avery.

Di Battista, A., Godfrey, C., Soo, C., Catroppa, C., & Anderson, V. (2014). Depression and health related quality of life in adolescent survivors of a traumatic brain injury: A pilot study. *PLoS One, 9*(7). https://doi.org/10.1371/journal.pone.0101842

Di Battista, A., Soo, C., Catroppa, C., & Anderson, V. (2012). Quality of life in children and adolescents post-TBI: A systematic review and meta-analysis. *Journal of Neurotrauma, 29*(9), 1717–1727.

Dodson, M. B. (2010). A model to guide the rehabilitation of high-functioning employees after mild brain injury. *Work, 36*(4), 449–457.

Douglas, J. M., Bracy, C. A., & Snow, P. C. (2016). Return to work and social communication ability following severe traumatic brain injury. *Journal of Speech, Language, and Hearing Research, 59*(3), 511–520.

Dunn, D. S., & Elliott, T. R. (2008). The place and promise of theory in rehabilitation psychology. *Rehabilitation Psychology, 53*(3), 254–267.

Elliott, R., Bohart, A. C., Watson, J. C., & Murphy, D. (2018). Therapist empathy and client outcome: An updated meta-analysis. *Psychotherapy, 55*(4), 399–410.

Ewing-Cobbs, L., Prasad, M. R., Swank, P., Kramer, L., Cox, C. S. Jr., Fletcher, J. M. . . . . Hasan, K. M. (2008). Arrested development and disrupted callosal microstructure following pediatric traumatic brain injury: Relation to neurobehavioral outcomes. *NeuroImage, 42*(4), 1305–1315.

Fang, Y., Mpofu, E., & Athanasou, J. (2017). Reducing depressive or anxiety symptoms in post-stroke patients: Pilot trial of a constructive integrative psychosocial intervention. *International Journal of Health Sciences, 11*(4), 53–58.

Fuchs, T. (2007). Psychotherapy of the lived space: A phenomenological and ecological concept. *American Journal of Psychotherapy, 61*(4), 423–439.

Gabbe, B. J., Brooks, C., Demmler, J. C., Macey, S., Hyatt, M. A., & Lyons, R. A. (2014). The association between hospitalisation for childhood head injury and academic performance: Evidence from a population e-cohort study. *Journal of Epidemiology & Community Health, 68*(5) 466–470.

Goldstein, K. (1952). The effect of brain damage on the personality. *Psychiatry, 15*(3), 245–260.

Hayes, S. C., Strosahl, K. D., & Wilson, K. G. (2003). *Acceptance and commitment therapy: An experiential approach to behavior change.* New York: Guilford Press.

Kabat-Zinn, J. (2013). *Full catastrophe living: Using the wisdom of your body and mind to face stress, pain, and illness* (revised and updated ed.). New York: Bantam Books.

Kauffman, J. (Ed.). (2002). *Loss of the assumptive world: A theory of traumatic loss.* New York: Brunner-Routledge.

Klonoff, P. S. (2010). *Psychotherapy after brain injury: Principles and techniques.* New York: Guilford Press.

Klonoff, P. S. (2011). A therapist experiential model of treatment for brain injury. *Bulletin of the Menninger Clinic, 75*(1), 21–42.

Klonoff, P. S. (2014). *Psychotherapy for families after brain injury.* New York: Springer Science + Business Media.

Klonoff, P. S., Olson, K. C., Talley, M. C., Husk, K. L., Myles, S. M., Gehrels, J., & Dawson, L. K. (2010). The relationship of cognitive retraining to neurological patients' driving status: The role of process variables and compensation training. *Brain Injury, 24*(2), 63–73.

Kohut, H. (1984). The curative effect of analysis: A preliminary statement based on the findings of self psychology. In A. Goldberg & P. E. Stepansky (Eds.), *How does analysis cure?* (pp. 64–79). Chicago, IL: University of Chicago Press.

Kreutzer, J. S., Marwitz, J. H., Godwin, E. E., & Arango-Lasprilla, J. C. (2010). Practical approaches to effective family intervention after brain injury. *Journal of Head Trauma Rehabilitation, 25*(2), 113–120.

Lanham, R. A., & Misukanis, T. (1999, Summer). Estimating premorbid intelligence: Determining change in cognition following brain injury. *Brain Injury Source, Pediatric Issue, 3*(3).

Lapsley, D., & Carlo, G. (2014). Moral development at the crossroads: New trends and possible futures. *Developmental Psychology, 50*(1), 1–7.

Lezak, M. D., Howieson, D. B., Loring, D. W., Hannay, H. J., & Fischer, J. S. (2004). *Neuropsychological assessment.* New York: Oxford University Press.

Li, L., & Liu, J. (2012). The effect of pediatric traumatic brain injury on behavioral outcomes: A systematic review. *Developmental Medicine & Child Neurology, 55*(1), 37–45.

Marazziti, D., Baroni, S., Landi, P., Ceresoli, D., & Dell'Osso, L. (2013). The neurobiology of moral sense: Facts or hypotheses? *Annals of General Psychiatry, 12*(1). https://doi.org/10.1186/1744-859X-12-6.

Martelli, M. F., Zasler, N. D., & Tiernan, P. (2012). Community based rehabilitation: Special issues. *NeuroRehabilitation, 31*(1), 3–18.

Mendez, M. F. (2009). The neurobiology of moral behavior: Review and neuropsychiatric implications. *CNS Spectrums, 14*(11), 608–620.

Norcross, J. C., & Goldfried, M. R. (2005). *Handbook of psychotherapy integration* (2nd ed.). New York: Oxford University Press.

Pascual, L., Rodrigues, P., & Gallardo-Pujol, D. (2013). How does morality work in the brain? A functional and structural perspective of moral behavior. *Frontiers in Integrative Neuroscience, 7*(65), https://doi.org/10.3389/fnint.2013.00065

Pollak, S. M., Pedulla, T., & Siegel, R. D. (2016). *Sitting together: Essential skills for mindfulness-based psychotherapy.* New York: Guilford Press.

Roos, S. (2002). *Chronic sorrow: A living loss.* New York: Brunner-Routledge.

Rosema, S., Crowe, L., & Anderson, V. (2012). Social function in children and adolescents after traumatic brain injury: A systemic review 1989–2011. *Journal of Neurotrauma, 29*(7), 1277–1291.

Rosema, S., Muscara, F., Anderson, V., Godfrey, C., Hearps, S., & Catroppa, C. (2015). The trajectory of long-term psychosocial development 16 years following childhood traumatic brain injury. *Journal of Neurotrauma, 32*(13), 976–983.

Ruff, R. M., & Chester, S. K. (2014). *Effective psychotherapy for individuals with brain injury.* New York: Guilford Press.

Ryan, N. P., Anderson, V., Godfrey, C., Eren, S., Rosema, S., Taylor, K., & Catroppa, C. (2013). Social communication mediates the relationship between emotion perception and externalizing behaviors in young adult survivors of pediatric traumatic brain injury. *International Journal of Developmental Neuroscience, 31*(8), 811–819.

Sandberg, S., & Grant, A. (2017). *Option B: Facing adversity, building resilience, and finding joy.* New York: Alfred A. Knopf.

Schachar, R. J., Park, L. S., & Dennis, M. (2015). Mental health implications of Traumatic Brain Injury (TBI) in children and youth. *Journal of the Canadian Academy of Child and Adolescent Psychiatry, 24*(2), 100–108.

Schönberger, M., Humle, F., & Teasdale, T. W. (2006). Subjective outcome of brain injury rehabilitation in relation to the therapeutic working alliance, client compliance and awareness. *Brain Injury, 20*(12), 1271–1282.

Taber-Thomas, B. C., Asp, E. W., Koenigs, M., Sutterer, M., Anderson, S. W., & Tranel, D. (2014). Arrested development: Early prefrontal lesions impair the maturation of moral judgement. *Brain: A Journal of Neurology, 137,* 1254–1261.

Tomaszewski, W., Buliński, L., Mirski, A., Rasmus, A., Kowalczyk, J., Bazan, M., & Pąchalska, M. (2014). An evaluation of antisocial behavior in children after traumatic brain injury: The prospect of improving the quality of life in rehabilitation. *Annals of Agricultural and Environmental Medicine, 21*(3), 649–653.

Vestri, A., Peruch, F., Marchi, S., Frare, M., Guerra, P., Pizzighello, S. . . . Martinuzzi, A. (2014). Individual and group treatment for patients with acquired brain injury in comprehensive rehabilitation. *Brain Injury, 28*(8), 1102–1108.

Wiart, L., Luauté, J., Stefan, A., Plantier, D., & Hamonet, J. (2016). Non pharmacological treatments for psychological and behavioural disorders following traumatic brain injury (TBI). A systematic literature review and expert opinion leading to recommendations. *Annals of Physical and Rehabilitation Medicine, 59*(1), 31–41.

Winson, R., Wilson, B. A., & Bateman, A. (Eds.). (2017). *The brain injury rehabilitation workbook.* New York: Guilford Press.

Wolf, E. S. (1988). *Treating the self: Elements of clinical self psychology.* New York: Guilford Press.

Worden, J. W. (2009). *Grief counselling and grief therapy: A handbook for the mental health practitioner.* New York: Springer.

Yalom, I. D. (2002). *The gift of therapy: An open letter to a new generation of therapists and their patients.* New York: HarperCollins Publishers.

Zarbo, C., Tasca, G. A., Cattafi, F., & Compare, A. (2016). Integrative psychotherapy works. *Frontiers in Psychology, 6,* 2021.

INDEX

Note: Page numbers in *italics* and **bold** indicate Figures and Tables, respectively.

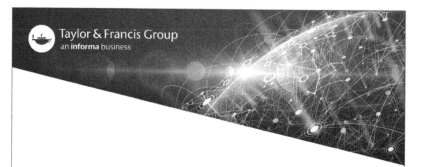

Printed in the United States
by Baker & Taylor Publisher Services